Dicing with Death
Chance, Risk and Health

Statisticians are engaged in an exhausting but exhilarating struggle with the biggest challenge that philosophy makes to science: how do we translate information into knowledge? Statistics tells us how to evaluate evidence, how to design experiments, how to turn data into decisions, how much credence should be given to whom to what and why, how to reckon chances and when to take them. Statistics deals with the very essence of the universe: chance and contingency are its discourse and statisticians know the vocabulary. If you think that statistics has nothing to say about what you do or how you could do it better, then you are either wrong or in need of a more interesting job. Stephen Senn explains here how statistics determines many decisions about medical care, from allocating resources for health, to determining which drugs to license, to cause-and-effect in relation to disease. He tackles big themes: clinical trials and the development of medicines, life tables, vaccines and their risks or lack of them, smoking and lung cancer and even the power of prayer. He entertains with puzzles and paradoxes and covers the lives of famous statistical pioneers. By the end of the book the reader will see how reasoning with probability is essential to making rational decisions in medicine, and how and when it can guide us when faced with choices that impact on our health and even life.

Dicing with Death

Chance, Risk and Health

STEPHEN SENN
University College London

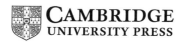
CAMBRIDGE
UNIVERSITY PRESS

PUBLISHED BY THE PRESS SYNDICATE OF THE UNIVERSITY OF CAMBRIDGE
The Pitt Building, Trumpington Street, Cambridge, United Kingdom

CAMBRIDGE UNIVERSITY PRESS
The Edinburgh Building, Cambridge, CB2 2RU, UK
40 West 20th Street, New York NY 10011–4211, USA
477 Williamstown Road, Port Melbourne, VIC 3207, Australia
Ruiz de Alarcón 13, 28014 Madrid, Spain
Dock House, The Waterfront, Cape Town 8001, South Africa

http://www.cambridge.org

First published 2003

Printed in the United Kingdom at the University Press, Cambridge

Typeface Lexicon No. 2 9/13 pt. and Lexicon No. 1   *System* LaTeX 2_ε [TB]

A catalogue record for this book is available from the British Library

Library of Congress Cataloguing in Publication data
Senn, Stephen.
  Dicing with death : chance, risk and health / Stephen Senn.
    p. cm.
  Includes bibliographical references and index.
  ISBN 0 521 83259 4 – ISBN 0 521 54023 2 (paperback)
  1. Medical statistics. 2. Medicine – Philosophy. 3. Medical care – Statistical
methods. I. Title.
  RA407.S46 2003 610′.7′27 – dc21   2003053199

ISBN 0 521 83259 4 hardback
ISBN 0 521 54023 2 paperback

The publisher has used its best endeavours to ensure that the URLs for external
websites referred to in this book are correct and active at the time of going to press.
However, the publisher has no responsibility for the websites and can make no
guarantee that a site will remain live or that the content is or will remain
appropriate.

For Victoria, Helen and Mark

... the twain were casting dice
'The game is done! I've won! I've won!'
Quoth she and whistles thrice.
    Coleridge, *The Rime of the Ancient Mariner*

Contents

Preface

Statistics is dull but disreputable, prosaic but misleading. Statisticians are the auditors of research: negative and uncreative book-keepers. If mathematics is the handmaiden of science, statistics is its whore: all that scientists are looking for is a quick fix without the encumbrance of a meaningful relationship. Statisticians are second-class mathematicians, third-rate scientists and fourth-rate thinkers. They are the hyenas, jackals and vultures of the scientific ecology: picking over the bones and carcasses of the game that the big cats, the biologists, the physicists and the chemists, have brought down.

Statistics is a wonderful discipline. It has it all: mathematics and philosophy, analysis and empiricism, as well as applicability, relevance and the fascination of data. It demands clear thinking, good judgement and flair. Statisticians are engaged in an exhausting but exhilarating struggle with the biggest challenge that philosophy makes to science: how do we translate information into knowledge? Statistics tells us how to evaluate evidence, how to design experiments, how to turn data into decisions, how much credence should be given to whom to what and why, how to reckon chances and when to take them. Statistics deals with the very essence of the universe: chance and contingency are its discourse and statisticians know the vocabulary. If you think that statistics has nothing to say about what you do or how you could do it better, then you are either wrong or in need of a more interesting job.

If you tend to the first of these views, this book is written to persuade you of the truth of the second and if you already accept the second it is here to confirm your faith. Statistics is all-pervading in science but it is also misunderstood. The non-scientist in the street probably has a clearer notion of physics, chemistry and biology than of statistics, regarding statisticians as numerical philatelists, mere collectors of numbers. The truth must out, and I am determined to out it and this book is how I have chosen to reveal it, but in a book like this it would be impossible to tell it all. Even within my own field of application, medical statistics, I cannot do that. There are many matters I should like to have covered but have not: the logic, or otherwise, of screening for disease, the use of statistics in health-care planning, statistical approaches to the creation of expert systems for diagnosis, the wonderful science of decision analysis and its application to selecting which drugs to develop, the world of sample surveys, the mathematics of genetics, the statistical approach to quality control and its application to monitoring surgery, the interpretation of hospital league tables, sequential analysis and the design of experiments.

Nevertheless, we shall cover some important matters: paradoxes in probability, significance tests, clinical trials, the Bayesian and frequentist schools of inference, the generalisability of results, the safety, or otherwise, of medicines and tobacco, life-tables and survival analysis, the summarising of evidence, the mathematics of measles, and even the application of statistics to the law. (If the relevance of the last of these to medical statistics is not clear, all will be revealed in Chapter 10.) Naturally I am convinced that this is all good stuff but some of it, I know, is strong medicine. I have tried to sugar the pill by coating the numerical with the biographical. We shall discuss not just statistics the subject but the statisticians who created it and a curious lot they turn out to be. We shall also, occasionally, take some strange diversions and the medically qualified reader may detect the symptoms of *knight's-move thought* (kmt) and conclude that the author is schizophrenic. (It must surely have been someone with kmt who first called it kmt.) But despite these diversions, whether biographical or otherwise, the numerical cannot be entirely avoided. I have helped the reader to spot it by spotting it myself, or at least starring it. There are two starred chapters, and these are more demanding than the rest. They can safely be omitted by those who find the mathematics off-putting, although, of course, I would not have included them if I had not felt that they were worth the struggle. A star attached to a section within a chapter also indicates more difficult material that can be skipped. A starred section within a starred chapter is for the top of the class.

I make no claims to omniscience. Statistics is the science of inference, the science of inference *for* science, and the defining characteristic of science is not its infallibility but its self-correcting ability. Some of what I say will need correcting. Although I have done some original historical research myself, this is limited to the first half of the last century and even there it is limited to a small part of the story. Elsewhere I have relied extensively on secondary sources, in particular the magnificent books by Anders Hald and Stephen Stigler.[1] Other sources are indicated in the footnotes to the chapters. I have also strayed into areas in which I have no particular expertise, the modelling of infectious diseases and statistics applied to the Law, for example. The subject is so vast that nobody can be expert in all aspects of it. My own personal research is mainly in the design and analysis of clinical trials but the book needed more than just that to give it wings.

I have many debts to acknowledge. Doris Altmann, Klaus Dietz, Paddy Farrington, Joe Gani, John Hayward and Jonathan Koehler provided me with copies of their papers. Abelard, Tom Boyd, Damien Defawe, Douglas Fleming, Marta Gacic-Dobo, Richard Greenway, Gerard Michon, Kenneth Milslead, Jane Oakley, Heikki Peltola, Belinda Thornton and Isabel Trevenna helped me obtain papers of others or provided me with data or information. David Brunnen, Iain Chalmers, Giovanni Della Cioppa, Paul Greenwood, Valerie Isham, Martin Jarvis, Geoff Paddle, Mervyn Stone and my daughter, Helen, provided helpful comments on various chapters. The book was submitted for the Wellcome Prize and was a runner up in 2002 and I am grateful to Sarah Bronsdon of the Wellcome Foundation for her encouragement. I am also most grateful to David Tranah of Cambridge University Press for welcoming the completed book with enthusiasm and to Sarah Price for her expert help in editing. Finally, I should like to thank my wife Victoria for persuading me to write it.

So, on with the book. I am going to try and convince you that when it comes to making decisions and scientific inferences, if you can't count you don't count. Let us roll the first die.

---

[1] A. Hald, *A History of Probability and Statistics and Their Applications before 1750*. John Wiley & Sons Ltd, 1990; A. Hald, *A History of Mathematical Statistics from 1750 to 1930*. John Wiley & sons Ltd, 1998; S. M. Stigler, *The History of Statistics: The Measurement of Uncertainty before 1900*. Belknap Press, 1986.

Permissions

The following are gratefully acknowledged for permission to cite from the following works. James Kirkup: *For the 90th Birthday of Sibelius* by James Kirkup. Howard Jacobson: *Coming from Behind* by Howard Jacobson, Vintage. The Random House Group Limited and Penguin Putnam Inc: Thomas Pynchon's *Gravity's Rainbow*, Jonathan Cape/Vintage. The Royal Society of Medicine: *Effectiveness and Efficiency* by Archie Cochrane, RSM Press. AP Watt Ltd on behalf of the estate of Jocelyn Hale and Teresa Elizabeth Perkins: *Uncommon Law* by AP Herbert. DEP International: *1 in 10* by UB40. Frederick C Crews and Penguin Putnam Inc: *The Pooh Perplex* by Fredrick C Crews. Harper Collins: *The Phantom Tollbooth* by Norton Juster, *Cheaper by the Dozen* by Frank B Gilbreth and Ernestine Gilbreth Carey and *The Book of Ebenezer Le Page* by GB Edwards. Harcourt Inc: *Arrowsmith* by Sinclair Lewis. The Arthur Ransome Literary Estate: *Winter Holiday* by Arthur Ransome. Cannongate books: *Naive Super* by Erland Loe, first published in Great Britain by Canongate Books Ltd, 14 High Street Edinburgh, EH1 1TE. Universal Music Publishing Group: *American Pie* by Don MacLean. Stranger Music and Sony Music: *Everybody Knows* by Leonard Cohen.

Circling the square

It's my bad friend Kent . . . Kent works at the Central Statistics Bureau. He knows how many litres of milk Norwegians drink per annum and how often people have sex. On average that is.

Erlend Loe, Naïve. Super

The charisma casualty. A scientist in need of an apology and the question he dreads

Look at that miserable student in the corner at the party. He could be my younger self. He was doing well until she asked the dreaded question. 'What are you studying?' At such a moment what would one not give for the right to a romantic answer: 'Russian,' perhaps or 'drama'. Or a coldly cerebral one: 'philosophy' or 'mathematics' or even 'physics'. Or to pass oneself as a modern Victor Frankenstein, a genetic engineer or a biochemist. That is where the action will be in this millennium. But statistics? It's like Kenny Everett's joke about elderly women: just like Australia, everyone knows where it is but no one wants to go there. Except that people do want to go to Australia.

Some years ago there was an advert for a French film, *Tatie Danielle*, about a misanthropic, manipulative and downright nasty old lady which ran, 'you don't know her, but she loathes you already'. Of most people one might just as well say, 'you've never studied statistics but you loathe it already'. You know already what it will involve (so many tonnes of coal mined in Silesia in 1963, so many deaths from TB in China in 1978). Well you are wrong. It has nothing, or hardly anything, to do with that. And if you have encountered it as part of some degree course, for no scientist or social scientist escapes, then you know that it consists of a number of algorithms to carry out tests of significance using data. Well you are also wrong. Statistics, like Bill Shankly's football, is not just a matter of life and death. 'Son, it's much more important than that.'

Statistics are and statistics is

Statistics singular, contrary to the popular perception, is not really about facts; it is about how we know, or suspect, or believe, that something is a fact. Because knowing about things involves counting and measuring them, then, it is true, that statistics plural are part of the concern of statistics singular, which is the science of quantitative reasoning. This science has much more in common with philosophy (in particular epistemology) than it does with accounting. Statisticians are applied philosophers. Philosophers argue how many angels can dance on the head of a needle; statisticians *count* them.

Or rather, count how many can *probably* dance. Probability is the heart of the matter, the heart of all matter if the quantum physicists can be believed. As far as the statistician is concerned this is true, whether the world is strictly deterministic as Einstein believed or whether there is a residual ineluctable indeterminacy. We can predict nothing with certainty but we can predict how uncertain our predictions will be, on average that is. Statistics is the science that tells us how.

Quacks and squares

I want to explain how important statistics is. For example, take my own particular field of interest, pharmaceutical clinical trials: experiments on human beings to establish the effects of drugs. Why, as a statistician, do I do research in this area? I don't treat patients. I don't design drugs. I scarcely know a stethoscope from a thermometer. I have forgotten most of the chemistry I ever knew and I never studied biology. But I have successfully designed and analysed clinical trials for a living. Why should it be that the International Conference on Harmonisations guidelines for Good Clinical Practice, the framework for the conduct of pharmaceutical trials in Europe, America and Japan should state, 'The sponsor should utilize qualified individuals (e.g. biostatisticians, clinical pharmacologists, and physicians) as appropriate, throughout all stages of the trial process, from designing the protocol and CRFs and planning the analyses to analyzing and preparing interim and final clinical trial reports.[1]'? We know why we need quacks but these 'squares' who go around counting things, what use are they? We don't treat patients with statistics do we?

High anxiety

Of course not. Suppose that you have just suffered a collapsed lung at 35 000 ft and, the cabin crew having appealed for help, a 'doctor' turns up. A Ph.D. in statistics would be as much use as a spare statistician at a party. You damn well want the doctor to be a medic. In fact this is precisely what happened to a lady travelling from Hong Kong to Britain in May 1995. She had fallen off a motorcycle on her way to the airport and had not realised the gravity of her injuries until airborne. Luckily for her, two resourceful physicians, Professor Angus Wallace and Dr. Tom Wang, were on board.[2] Initially distracted by the pain she was experiencing in her arm, they eventually realised that she had a more serious problem. She had, in fact, a 'tension pneumothorax', a life-threatening condition that required immediate attention. With the help of the limited medical equipment on board plus a coat hanger and a bottle of Evian water the two doctors performed an emergency operation to release air from her pleural cavity and restore her ability to breathe normally. The operation was a complete success and the woman recovered rapidly.

This story illustrates the very best aspects of the medical profession and why we value its members so highly. The two doctors concerned had to react quickly to a rapidly developing emergency, undertake a technical manoeuvre in which they were probably not specialised and call not only on their medical knowledge but on that of physics as well: the bottle of water was used to create a water seal. There is another evidential lesson for us here, however. We are convinced by the story that the intervention was necessary and successful. This is a very reasonable conclusion. Amongst factors that make it reasonable are that the woman's condition was worsening rapidly and that within a few minutes of the operation her condition was reversed.

A chronic problem

However, much of medicine is not like that. General practitioners, for example, busy and harassed as they are typically have little chance of learning the effect of the treatments they employ. This is because most of what is done is either for chronically ill patients for whom no rapid reversal can be expected or for patients who are temporarily ill, looking for some relief or a speedier recovery and who will not report back. Furthermore, so short is the half-life of relevance of medicine that if (s)he is middle-aged, half of what (s)he learned at university will now be regarded as outmoded if not downright wrong.

The trouble with medical education is that it prepares doctors to learn facts, whereas really what the physician needs is a strategy for learning. The joke (not mine) is that three students are asked to memorise the telephone directory. The mathematician says, 'why?', the lawyer says, 'how long have I got?' and the medical student says, 'will the Yellow Pages also be in the exam?' This is changing, however. There is a new movement for evidence-based medicine that stresses the need for doctors to remain continually in touch with developments in treatment and also to assess the evidence for such new treatment critically. Such evidence will be quantitative. Thus doctors are going to have to learn more about statistics.

It would be wrong, however, to give the impression that there is an essential antagonism between medicine and statistics. In fact the medical profession has made important contributions to the theory of statistics. As we shall see when we come to consider John Arbuthnot, Daniel Bernoulli and several other key figures in the history of statistics, many who contributed had had a medical education, and in the medical specialty of epidemiology many practitioners can be found who have made important contributions to statistical theory. However, on the whole, it can be claimed that these contributions have arisen because the physician has come to think like a statistician: with scepticism. 'This is plausible, how might it be wrong?' could be the statistician's catch-phrase. In the sections that follow, we consider some illustrative paradoxes.

A familiar familial fallacy?

'Mr Brown has exactly two children. At least one of them is a boy. What is the probability that the other is a girl?' What could be simpler than that? After all, the other child either is or is not a girl. I regularly use this example on the statistics courses I give to life scientists working in the pharmaceutical industry. They all agree that the probability is one-half.

So they are all wrong. I haven't said that the *older* child is a boy. The child I mentioned, the boy, could be the older or the younger child. This means that Mr Brown can have one of three possible combinations of two children: both boys, elder boy and younger girl, elder girl and younger boy, the fourth combination of two girls being excluded by what I have stated.

But of the three combinations, in two cases the other child is a girl so that the requisite probability is $^2/_3$. This is illustrated as follows.

	Possible	Possible	Possible	Excluded
Elder	♂	♂	♀	♀
Younger	♂	♀	♂	♀

This example is typical of many simple paradoxes in probability: the answer is easy to explain but nobody believes the explanation. However, the solution I have given *is* correct.

Or is it? That was spoken like a probabilist. A probabilist is a sort of mathematician. He or she deals with artificial examples and logical connections but feel no obligation to say anything about the real world. My demonstration, however, relied on the assumption that the three combinations boy–boy, boy–girl and girl–boy are equally likely and this may not be true. The difference between a statistician and a probabilist is that the latter will define the problem so that this is true, whereas the former will consider *whether* it is true and obtain data to test its truth.

Suppose we make the following assumptions: (1) the sex ratio at birth is 50:50; (2) there is no tendency for boys or girls to run in a given family; (3) the death rates in early years of life are similar for both sexes; (4) parents do not make decisions to stop or continue having children based on the mix of sexes they already have; (5) we can ignore the problem of twins. Then the solution is reasonable. (Provided there is nothing else I have overlooked!) However, the first assumption is known to be false, as we shall see in the next chapter. The second assumption is believed to be (approximately) true but this belief is based on observation and analysis; there is nothing logically inevitable about it. The third assumption is false, although in economically developed societies, the disparity in the death rates between sexes, although considerable in later life, is not great before adulthood. There is good evidence that the fourth assumption is false. The fifth is not completely ignorable, since some children are twins, some twins are identical and all identical twins are of the same sex. We now consider a data set that will help us to check our answer.

In an article in the magazine *Chance*, in 2001, Joseph Lee Rogers and Debby Doughty attempt to answer the question, 'Does having boys or girls run in the family?'.[3] The conclusion that they come to is that it does not, or at least, if it does that the tendency is at best very weak. To establish this conclusion they use data from an American study, the National

Longitudinal Survey of Youth (NLSY). This originally obtained a sample of over 12 000 respondents aged 14–21 years in 1979. The NLSY sample has been followed up from time to time since. Rogers and Doughty use data obtained in 1994, by which time the respondents were aged 29–36 years and had had 15 000 children between them. The same data that they use to investigate the sex distribution of families can be used to answer our question.

Of the 6089 NLSY respondents who had had at least one child, 2444 had had exactly two children. In these 2444 families the distribution of children was boy–boy, 582, girl–girl, 530, boy–girl 666 and girl–boy, 666. If we exclude girl–girl, the combination that is excluded by the question, then we are left with 1914 families. Of these families 666 + 666 = 1332 had one boy and one girl so that the proportion of families with at least one boy in which the other child is a girl is 1332/1914 $\simeq$ 0.70. So, in fact, our requisite probability is not $^2/_3$ as we previously suggested but $^7/_{10}$ (approximately).

Or is it? We have moved from a view of probability that tries to identify equally probable cases, what is sometimes called classical probability, to one that uses relative frequencies. There are, however, several objections to using this ratio as a probability, of which two are particularly important. The first is that a little reflection shows that it is obvious that such a ratio is itself subject to chance variation. To take a simple example, even if we believe a die to be fair we would not expect that whenever we rolled the die six times we would obtain exactly one 1, 2, 3, 4, 5 & 6. The second objection is that even if this ratio is an adequate approximation to some probability, why should we accept that it is the probability that applies to Mr Brown? After all, I have not said that he is either an American citizen who was aged 14–21 in 1971 or has had children with such a person, yet this is the group from which the ratio was obtained.

The first objection might lead me to prefer a theoretical value such as the $^2/_3$ obtained by our first argument to the value of approximately $^7/_{10}$ (which is of course very close to it) obtained by the second. In fact, statisticians have developed a number of techniques for deciding how reasonable such a theoretical value is.

A likely tale*

One method is due to the great British statistician and geneticist R. A. Fisher (1890–1962) whom we shall encounter again in various chapters in this book. This is based on his idea of likelihood. What you can do in a circumstance like this, he points out, is to investigate each and every possible value for the probability from 0 to 1. You can then try each of these values in turn and see how likely the data are given the value of the probability you currently assume. The data for this purpose are that of the 1914 relevant families: in 1332 the other child was a girl and in 582 it was a boy. Let the probability in a given two-child family that the other child is a girl where at least one child is male be P, where, for example, P might be $2/3$ or $7/10$ or indeed any value we wish to investigate. Suppose that we go through the 1914 family records one by one. The probability of any given record corresponding to a mixed-sex family is P and the probability of it corresponding to a boys only family is $(1-P)$. Suppose that we observe that the first 1332 families are mixed sex and the next 582 are boys only. The likelihood, to use Fisher's term, of this occurring is $P \times P \times P \cdots P$, where there are 1332 such terms P, multiplied by $(1-P) \times (1-P) \times (1-P) \cdots (1-P)$, where there are 582 such terms. Using the symbol L for likelihood, we may write this as

$$L = P^{1332}(1-P)^{582}.$$

Now, of course, we have not seen the data in this particular order; in fact, we know nothing about the order at all. However, the likelihood we have calculated is the same for any given order so that all we need to do is multiply it by the number of orders (sequences) in which the data could occur. This turns out to be quite unnecessary, however, since whatever the value of P, whether $2/3$, $7/10$ or some other value, the number of possible sequences is the same so that in each of such cases the number we would multiply L by would be the same. This number is thus irrelevant to our inferences about P and, indeed, for any two values of P, the ratio of the two corresponding values of L does not depend on the number of ways in which we can obtain 1332 mixed-sex and 582 two-boy families.

It turns out that the value of P that maximises L is that which is given by our empirical proportion so that we may write $P_{max} = 1332/1914$. We can now express the likelihood, L, of any value of P as a ratio of the likelihood L_{max} corresponding to P_{max}. This has been done and plotted against all possible values of P in the Figure 1.1. One can see that this ratio reaches a maximum one at the observed proportion, indicated by a solid line, and tails off rapidly either side. In fact, for our theoretical answer of $2/3$, indicated by the dashed line, the ratio is less than $1/42$. Thus the observed

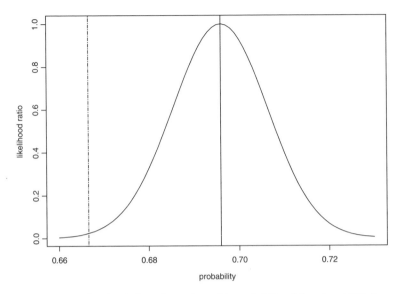

Figure 1.1 Likelihood ratio for various values of the probability of the other child being a girl given the NLSY sample data.

proportion is 42 times more likely to occur if the true probability is $P_{max} = 1332/1914$ than if it is the theoretical value of $^2/_3$ suggested.

An unlikely tail?

This is all very well but the reader will justifiably protest that the best fitting pattern will always fit the data better than some theory that issues a genuine prediction. For example, nobody would seriously maintain that the next time somebody obtains a sample of exactly 1914 persons having exactly two children, at least one of which is male, they will also observe that in 1332 cases the other is female. Another, perhaps not very different proportion would obtain and this other proportion would of course not only fit the data better than the theoretical probability of $^2/_3$, but it would also fit the data better than the proportion 1332/1914 previously observed.

In fact we have another data set with which we can check this proportion. This comes from the US Census Bureau National Interview Survey, a yearly random sample of families. Amongst the 342 018 households on which data were obtained from 1987 to 1993, there were 42 888 families with exactly two children, 33 365 with at least one boy. The split amongst the 33 365 was boy–girl, 11 118, girl–boy, 10 913 and boy–boy 11 334. Thus 22 031 of the families had one boy and one girl and the proportion we require is 22 031/33 365 $\simeq$ 0.66, which is closer to the theoretical value than our previous empirical answer. This suggests that we should not be too hasty in rejecting a plausible theoretical value in favour of some apparently better fitting alternative. How can we decide when to reject such a theoretical value?

This statistical problem of deciding when data should lead to rejection of a theory has a very long history and we shall look at attempts to solve it in the next chapter. Without entering into details here we consider briefly the approach of significance testing which, again, is particularly associated with Fisher, although it did not originate with him. This is to imagine for the moment that the theoretical value is correct and then pose the question, 'if the value is correct, how unusual are the data'.

Defining exactly what is meant by unusual turns out to be extremely controversial. One line of argument suggests, however, that if we were to reject the so-called null hypothesis that the true probability is $^2/_3$, then we have done so where the observed ratio is 1332/1914, which is higher than $^2/_3$, and would be honour bound to do so had the ratio been even higher. We thus calculate the probability of observing 1332 or more mixed-sex families when the true probability is $^2/_3$. This sort of probability is referred to as a 'tail-area' probability and, sparing the reader the details,[4] in this case it turns out to be 0.00337. However, we could argue that we would have been just as impressed by an observed proportion that was lower than the hypothesised value $^2/_3$ as by finding one that was higher, so that we ought to double this probability. If we do, we obtain a value of 0.0067. This sort of probability is referred to as a 'P-value' and is very commonly (many would say far too commonly) found in scientific, in particular medical, literature.

Should we reject or accept our hypothesised value? A conventional 'level of significance' often used is 5% or 0.05. If the P-value is lower than this the hypothesis in question is 'rejected', although it is generally admitted that this is a very weak standard of significance. If we reject $^2/_3$, however, what are we going to put in its place? As we have already argued it will be most unlikely for the true probability to be exactly equal to the observed proportion. That being so, might $^2/_3$ not be a better bet after all? We shall not pursue this here, however. Instead we now consider a more serious problem.

Right but irrelevant?

Why should we consider the probability we have been trying to estimate as being relevant to Mr Brown? There are all sorts of objections one could raise. Mr Brown might be British, for example, but our data come from an American cohort. Why should such data be relevant to the question? Also since Mr Brown's other child either is or is not a girl what on earth can it mean to speak of the probability of its being a girl.

This seemingly trivial difficulty turns out to be at the heart of a disagreement between two major schools of statistical inference, the frequentist and the Bayesian school, the latter being named after Thomas Bayes, 1701–1761, an English non-conformist minister whose famous theorem we shall meet in the next chapter.

The frequentist solution is to say that probabilities of single events are meaningless. We have to consider (potentially) infinite classes of events. Thus my original question is ill-posed and should perhaps have been, 'if we choose an individual at random and find that this individual is male and has two children at least one of which is male, what is the probability that the other is female?' We then can consider this event as one that is capable of repetition and the probability then becomes then long-run relative frequency with which the event occurs.

The Bayesian solution is radically different. This is to suggest that the probability in question is what you believe it to be since it represents your willingness to bet on the relevant event. You are thus free to declare it to be anything at all. For example, if you are still unconvinced by the theoretical arguments I have given and the data that have been presented that, whatever the probability is, it is much closer to $2/3$ than $1/2$, you are perfectly free to call the probability $1/2$ instead. However, be careful! Betting has consequences. If you believe that the probability is $1/2$ and are not persuaded by any evidence to the contrary, you might be prepared to offer odds of evens on the child being a boy. Suppose I offered to pay you £5 if the other child is a boy provided you paid me £4 if the child is a girl. You ought to accept the bet since the odds are more attractive than evens, which you regard as appropriate. If, however, we had played this game for each family you would have lost 1332×4 for only 582×5 gained and I would be £2418 better off at your expense![5]

We shall not pursue these discussions further now. However, some of these issues will reappear in later chapters and indeed from time to time throughout the book. Instead, we now present another paradox.

The Will Rogers phenomenon

A medical officer of public health keeps a track year by year of the perinatal mortality rate in his district for all births delivered at home and also for all those delivered at hospital using health service figures. (The perinatal mortality rate is the sum of stillbirths and deaths under one week of age divided by the total number of births, live and still, and is often used in public health as a measure of the outcome of pregnancy.) He notices, with satisfaction, a steady improvement year by year in both the hospital and the home rate.

However, as part of the general national vital registration system, corresponding figures are being obtained district by district, although not separately for home and hospital deliveries. By chance, a statistician involved in compiling the national figures and the medical officer meet at a function and start discussing perinatal mortality. The statistician is rather surprised to hear of the continual improvement in the local district since she knows that over the past decade there has been very little change nationally. Later she checks the figures for the medical officer's district and these confirm the general national picture. Over the last decade there has been little change.

In fact the medical officer is not wrong about the rates. He is wrong to be satisfied with his district's performance. He has fallen victim to what is sometimes called 'the stage migration phenomenon'. This was extensively described by the Yale-based epidemiologist Alvin Feinstein and colleagues in some papers in the mid 1980s.[6] They found improved survival stage by stage in groups of cancer patients but no improvement over all.

How can such phenomena be explained? Quite simply. By way of explanation, Feinstein et al. quote the American humorist Will Rogers who said that when the Okies left Oklahoma for California, the average intelligence was improved in two States. Imagine that the situation in the district in question is that most births deemed low risk take place at home and have done throughout the period in question and that most births deemed high risk take place in hospital and have done so throughout the period in question. There has been a gradual shift over the years of moderate-risk births from home to hospital. The result is a dilution of the high-risk births in hospital with moderate-risk cases. On the other hand, the home-based deliveries are becoming more and more tilted towards low risk. Consequently there is an improvement in both without any improvement over all.

The situation is illustrated in Figure 1.2 below. We have a mixture of o and X symbols on the sheet. The former predominate on the left and the latter on the right. A vertical line divides the sheet into two unequal regions. By moving the line to the right we will extend the domain of the left-hand region, adding more points. Since we will be adding

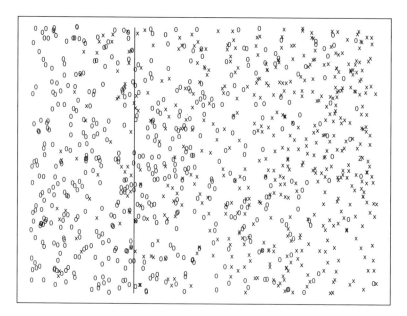

Figure 1.2 Illustration of the stage migration phenomenon.

regions in which there are relatively more and more X's than o's, we will be increasing the proportion of the former. However, simultaneously, we will be subtracting regions from the right-hand portion in which, relative to those that remain, there will be fewer X's than o's, hence we are also increasing the proportion of the former here.

Simpson's paradox[7]

The Will Rogers phenomenon is closely related to 'Simpson's paradox', named from a paper of 1951 by EH Simpson,[8] although described at least as early as 1899 by the British statistician Karl Pearson.'[9] This is best explained by example and we consider one presented by Julious and Mullee.[10] They give data for the Poole diabetic cohort in which patients are cross-classified by type of diabetes and as either dead or 'censored', which is to say, alive. The reason that the term 'censored' is used is that in the pessimistic vocabulary of survival-analysis, life is a temporary phenomenon and someone who is alive is simply not yet dead. What the statistician would like to know is how long he or she lived but this information is not (yet) available and so is censored. We shall look at survival analysis in more detail in Chapter 7.

Table 1.1. *Frequencies (percentages) of patients in the Poole diabetic cohort, cross-classified by type of diabetes and whether 'dead' or 'censored', i.e. alive.*

	Type of diabetes		
	Non-insulin dependent	Insulin dependent	
All Patients			
Censored	326(60)	253(71)	579
Dead	218(40)	105(29)	323
	544(100)	358(100)	902
Subjects aged ≤ 40			
Censored	15(100)	129(99)	144
Dead	0(0)	1(1)	1
	15(100)	130(100)	145
Subjects aged > 40			
Censored	311(59)	124(54)	435
Dead	218(41)	104(46)	322
	529(100)	228(100)	757

The data are given in Table 1.1 below in terms of frequencies (percentages) and show subjects dead or censored by type of diabetes. When age is not taken into account it turns out that a higher proportion of non-insulin dependent are dead (40%) than is the case for insulin-dependent diabetes (29%). However, when the subjects are stratified by age (40 and younger or over 40) then in both of the age groups the proportion dead is higher in the insulin-dependent group. Thus the paradox consists of observing that an association between two factors is reversed when a third is taken into account.

But is this really paradoxical? After all we are used to the fact that when making judgements about the influence of factors we must compare like with like. We all know that further evidence can overturn previous judgement. In the Welsh legend, the returning Llewelyn is met by his hound Gelert at the castle door. Its muzzle is flecked with blood. In the nursery the scene is one of savage disorder and the infant son is missing. Only once the hound has been put to the sword is the child heard to cry and discovered safe and sound by the body of a dead wolf. The additional evidence reverses everything: Llewelyn and not his hound is revealed as a faithless killer.

In our example the two groups are quite unlike and most commentators would agree that the more accurate message as regards the relative seriousness of insulin and non-insulin diabetes is given by the stratified approach, which is to say the approach that also takes account of the age of the patient. The fact that non-insulin diabetes develops on average at a much later age is muddying the waters.

Suppose that the numbers in the table remain the same but refer now to a clinical trial in some life-threatening condition and we replace 'Type of diabetes' by 'Treatment' and 'Non-insulin dependent' by 'A' and 'Insulin-dependent' by 'B' and 'Subjects' by 'Patients'. An incautious interpretation of the table would then lead us to a truly paradoxical conclusion. Treating young patients with A rather than B is beneficial (or at least not harmful – the numbers of deaths, o in the one case and 1 in the other, are very small). Treating older patients with A rather than B is beneficial. However, the overall effect of switching patients from B to A would be to increase deaths overall.

In his brilliant book, *Causality*, Judea Pearl gives Simpson's paradox pride of place.[11] Many statisticians have taken Simpson's paradox to mean that judgements of causality based on observational studies are ultimately doomed. We could never guarantee that further refined observation would not lead to a change in opinion. Pearl points out, however, that we are capable of distinguishing causality from association because there is a difference between seeing and doing. In the case of the trial above we may have seen that the trial is badly imbalanced but we know that the treatment given cannot affect the age of the patient at baseline, that is to say before the trial starts. However, age very plausibly will affect outcome and so it is a factor that should be accounted for of when judging the effect of treatment. If in future we change a patient's treatment we will not (at the moment we change it) change their age. So there is no paradox. We can improve the survival of both young and the old and will not, in acting in this way, adversely affect the survival of the population as a whole.

O. J. Simpson's paradox

The statistics demonstrate that only one-tenth of one percent of men who abuse their wives go on to murder them. And therefore it's very important for that fact to be put into empirical perspective, and for the jury not to be led to believe that a single instance, or two instances of alleged abuse necessarily means that the person then killed.

The statement was made on the Larry King show by a member of OJ Simpson's defence team.[12] No doubt he thought it was a relevant fact for the Jury to consider. However, the one thing that was not in dispute in this case was that Nicole Simpson had been murdered. She was murdered by somebody. If not by the man who had allegedly abused her then by someone else. Suppose now that we are looking at the case of a murdered woman who was in an abusive relationship and are considering the possibility that she was murdered by someone who was not her abusive partner. What is sauce for the goose is sauce for the gander: if the first probability was relevant so is this one. What is the probability that a woman who has been in an abusive relationship is murdered by someone other than her abuser? This might plausibly be less than one-tenth of one percent. After all, most women are not murdered.

And this, of course, is the point. The reason that the probability of an abusive man murdering his wife is so low is that the vast majority of women are not murdered and this applies also to women in an abusive relationship. But this aspect of the event's rarity, since the event has occurred, is not relevant. An unusual event has happened, whatever the explanation. The point is, rather, which of two explanations is more probable: murder by the alleged abuser or murder by someone else.

Two separate attempts were made to answer this question. We have not gone far enough yet into our investigation of probability to be able to explain how the figures were arrived at but merely quote the results. The famous Bayesian statistician Jack Good, writing in *Nature*, comes up with a probability of 0.5 that a previously abused murdered wife has been murdered by her husband.[13] Merz and Caulkins,[14] writing in *Chance*, come up with a figure of 0.8. These figures are in far from perfect agreement but serve, at least, to illustrate the irrelevance of 1 in 1000.

Tricky traffic

Figure 1.3 shows road accidents in Lothian region, Scotland, by site. It represents data from four years (1979–1982) for 3112 sites on a road network. For each site the number of accidents recorded are available on a yearly basis. The graph plots the mean accidents per site in the second two-year period as a function of the number of accidents in the first two-year period. For example, for all those sites that by definition had exactly two accidents over the first two-year period, the average number of accidents has been calculated over the second two-year period. This has also been done

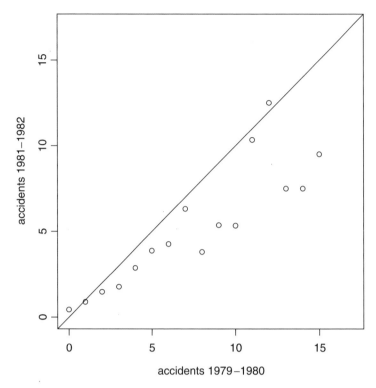

Figure 1.3 Accidents by road site, Lothian Region 1979–1982. Second two-year period plotted against first.

for those sites that had no accidents, as well as for those that had exactly one accident, and, continuing on the other end of the scale, for those that had three, four, etc. accidents.

The figure also includes a line of exact equality going through the points 1,1 and 2,2 and so forth. It is noticeable that most of the points lie to the right of the line of equality. It appears that road accidents are improving.

However, we should be careful. We have not treated the two periods identically. The first period is used to *define* the points (all sites that had exactly three accidents and so forth) whereas the second is simply used to *observe* them. Perhaps we should reverse the way that we look at accidents just to check and use the second period values to define our sites and the first period ones to observe them. This has been done in Figure 1.4. There is now a surprising result. Most of the points are still to the right of

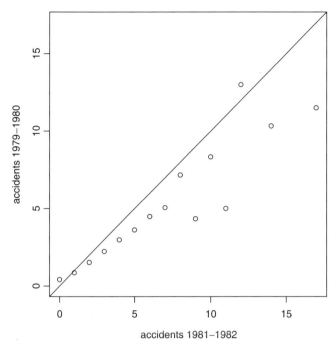

Figure 1.4 Accidents by road site, Lothian Region 1979–1982. First two-year period plotted against second.

the line, which is to say below the line of exact equality, but since the axes have changed this now means that the first-period values are higher than the second-period one. The accident rate is getting better.

The height of improbability

The data are correct. The explanation is due to a powerful statistical phenomenon called regression to the mean discovered by the Victorian scientist Francis Galton, whom we shall encounter again in Chapter 6. Obviously Galton did not have the Lothian road accident data! What he had were data on heights of parents and their adult offspring. Observing that women are on average 8% higher than men, he converted female heights to a male equivalent by multiplying by 1.08. Then, by calculating a 'mid-parent' height, the average of father's height and mother's adjusted height, he was able to relate the height of adult children to that of parents. He made a surprising discovery. If your parents were taller than average,

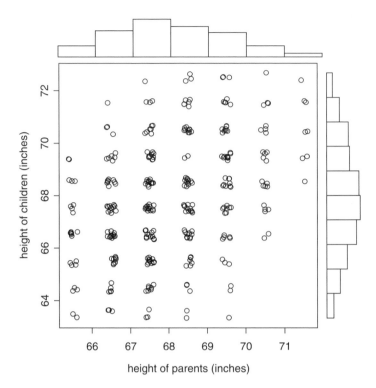

Figure 1.5 Galton' data. Heights of children in inches plotted against the adjusted average height of their parents.

although, unsurprisingly, you were likely to be taller than average, you were likely to be shorter than your parents. Similarly if your parents were shorter than average you were likely to be shorter than average but taller than your parents. Figure 1.5 below is a more modern representation of Galton's data, albeit very similar to the form he used himself.

The scatterplot in the middle plots children's heights against parents'. The lumpy appearance of the data is due to the fact that Galton records them to the nearest inch. Thus several points would appear on top of each other but for the fact that they have been 'jittered' here to separate them. The margins of the square have the plots for parents, heights irrespective of the height of children and vice-versa represented in the form of a 'histogram'. The areas of the bars of the histograms are proportional to the number of individuals in the given height group.

How can these phenomena be explained? We shall return to road accidents in a minute. Let us look at Galton's heights first of all. Suppose that it is the case that the distribution of height from generation to generation is stable. The mean is not changing and the spread of values is also not changing. Suppose also that there is not a perfect correlation between heights. This is itself a concept strongly associated with Galton. For our purposes we simply take this to mean that height of offspring cannot be perfectly predicted from height of parents – there is some variability in the result. Of course we know this to be true since, for example, brothers do not necessarily have identical heights. Now consider the shortest parents in a generation. If their children were on average of the same height, some would be taller but some would be shorter. Also consider the very tallest parents in a generation. If their offspring were on average as tall as them, some would be smaller but some would be taller. But this means that the spread of heights in the next generation would have to be greater than before, because the shortest members would now be shorter than the shortest before and the tallest would now be taller than the tallest before. But this violates what we have said about the distribution – that the spread is *not* increasing. In fact the only way that we can avoid the spread increasing is if *on average* the children of the shortest are taller than their parents and *if on average* the children of the tallest are shorter than their parents.

In actual fact, the discussion above is somewhat of a simplification. Even if variability of heights is not changing from generation to generation, whereas the heights of the children that are plotted are heights of individuals, the heights of the parents are (adjusted) averages of two individuals and this makes them less variable, as can be seen by studying Figure 1.5. However, it turns out that in this case the regression effect still applies.

Figure 1.6 is a mathematical fit to these data similar to the one that Galton found himself. It produces idealised curves representing our marginal plots above as well as some concentric contours representing greater and greater frequency of points in the scatterplot as one moves to the centre. The reader need not worry. We have no intention of explaining *how* to calculate this. It does, however, illustrate one part of the statistician's task – fitting mathematical (statistical) models to data. Also shown are the two lines, the so-called regression lines, that would give us the 'best' prediction of height of children from parents (solid) and parent's height from children (dashed) as well as the line of exact equality (dotted) that lies roughly between them both. (All three lines would meet at a point if the average height of children was exactly equal to the average for parents, but it is slightly different being 68.04 in inches in the one case and 67.92 in the other.) Note that since the regression line for children's heights as a function of parents' heights is less steep than the line

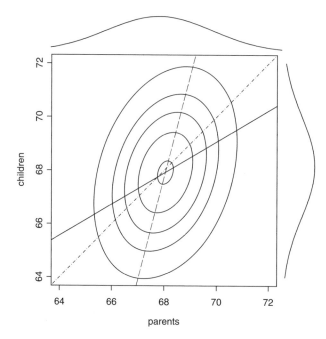

Figure 1.6 A bivariate normal distribution fitted to Galton's data showing also the line of equality and the two regression lines.

of exact equality, it will lead to predictions for the height of children that are closer to the mean than that of their parents. A corresponding effect is found with the other regression line. It is one of the extraordinary mysteries of statistics that the best prediction of parent's height from children's height is *not* given by using the line which provides the best prediction of children's heights from parent's heights.

Don't it make my brown eyes blue[15]

If this seems an illogical fact, it is none the less a fact of life. Let us give another example from genetics. Blue-eye colour is a so-called recessive characteristic. It thus follows that if any individual has blue eyes he or she must have two blue genes since, brown eye-colour being dominant, if the individual had one brown gene his or her eyes would be brown. Thus if we know that a child's biological parents both have blue eyes we can guess that the child must have blue eyes with probability almost one (barring mutations). On the other hand, a child with blue eyes could have one or even two parents with brown eyes since a brown-eyed parent can have a blue gene. Thus the probability of both parents having blue eyes is not one. The prediction in one direction is not the same as the prediction in the other.

Regression to the mean and the meaning of regression

Now return to the road accident data. The data are correct but one aspect of them is rather misleading. The points represent vastly different numbers of sites. In fact the most common number of accidents over any two-year period is zero. For example, in 1979–1980 out of 3112 sites in total, 1779 had no accidents at all. Furthermore the mean numbers of accidents for both two-year periods were very close to 1, being 0.98 in the first two-year period and 0.96 in the second. Now look at Figure 1.3 and the point corresponding to zero accidents in the first two-year period. That point is above the line and it is obvious that it has to be. The sites represented are those with a perfect record and since perfection cannot be guaranteed for ever, the mean for these sites was bound to increase. Some of the sites were bound to lose their perfect record and they would bring the mean up from zero which is what it was previously by definition, sites having been selected on this basis.

But if the best sites will deteriorate on average, then the worst will have to get better to maintain the average and this is exactly what we are observing. It just so happens that the mean value is roughly one accident per two years. The whole distribution is pivoting about this point. If we look at the higher end of the distribution, the reason for this phenomenon, which is nowadays termed 'regression to the mean', a term that Galton used interchangeably with, 'reversion to mediocrity', is that, although some of the sites included as bad have a true and genuine long-term bad record, some have simply been associated with a run of bad luck. On average the bad luck does not persist. Hence the record regresses to the mean.

Systolic magic

Regression to the mean is a powerful and widespread cause of spontaneous change where items or individuals have been selected for inclusion in a study because they are extreme. Since the phenomenon is puzzling, bewildering and hard to grasp we attempt one last demonstration: this time with a simulated set of blood pressure readings.

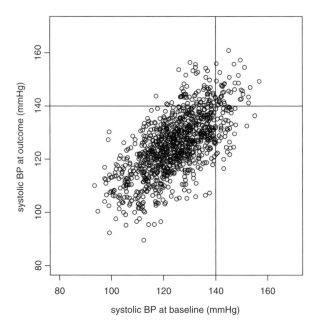

Figure 1.7 Systolic BP (mmHg) at baseline and outcome for 1000 individuals.

Figure 1.7 below gives systolic blood pressure reading in mmHg for a population of 1000 individuals. The data have been simulated so that the mean value at outcome and baseline is expected to be 125 mmHg. Those readers who have encountered the statistician's common measure of spread, the standard deviation, may like to note that this is 12 mmHg at outcome and baseline. Such readers will also have encountered the correlation coefficient. This is 0.7 for this example. Other readers should not worry about this but concentrate on the figure. The data are represented by the scatterplot and this is meant to show (1) that there is no real change between outcome and baseline, (2) that in general higher values at baseline are accompanied by higher values at outcome, but (3) this relationship is far from perfect.

Suppose that we accept that a systolic BP of more than 140 mmHg indicates hypertension. The vertical line on the graph indicates a boundary at baseline for this definition and the horizontal line a boundary at outcome. Making due allowances for random variation, there appears to be very little difference between the situation at baseline and outcome.

Suppose, however, we had decided not to follow the whole population but instead had merely followed up those whose baseline blood pressure

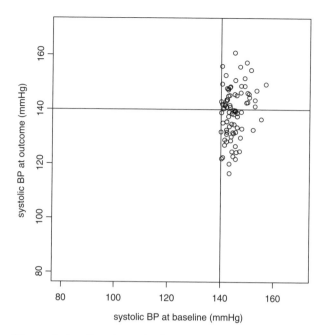

Figure 1.8 Systolic BP (mmHg) at baseline and outcome for a group of individuals selected because their baseline BP is in excess of 140 mmHg.

was in excess of 140 mmHg. The picture, as regards patients with readings at both baseline and outcome, would then be the one in Figure 1.8. But here we have a quite misleading situation. Some of the patients who had a reading in excess of 140 mmHg now have readings that are below. If we had the whole picture there would be a compensating set of readings for patients who were previously below the cut-off but are now above. But these are missing.

We thus see that regression to the mean is a powerful potential source of bias, particularly dangerous if we neglect to have a control group. Suppose, for example, that in testing the effect of a new drug we had decided to screen a group of patients only selecting those for treatment whose systolic blood pressure was in excess of 140 mmHg. We would see a spontaneous improvement whether or not the treatment was effective.

Paradoxical lessons?

The previous examples serve to make the point: statistics can be deceptively easy. Everybody believes they can understand and interpret them.

In practice, making sense of data can be difficult and one must take care in organising the circumstances for their collection if one wishes to come to a reasonable conclusion. For example, the puzzling, pervasive and apparently perverse phenomenon of regression to the mean is one amongst many reasons why the randomised clinical trial (RCT) has gained such popularity as a means to test the effects of medical innovation. If regression to the mean applies it will also affect the control group and this permits its biasing influence to be removed by comparison. There is no doubt that many were deceived by regression to the mean. Some continue to be so.

We hope that the point has been made in this chapter. Our 'square' has a justification for existence. Probability is subtle and data can deceive but how else are we to learn about the world except by observing it and what are observations when marshalled together but data? And who will take the time and care necessary to learn the craft of interpreting the data if not the statistician?

Wrapping up: the plan and the purpose

Medicine showed a remarkable development in the last century, not just in terms of the techniques that were developed for treating patients but also in the techniques that were developed for judging techniques. In the history of medicine, the initial conflict between the physician as professional and the physician as scientist meant that the science suffered. The variability of patients and disease, and the complexity of the human body made the development of scientific approaches difficult. Far more care had to be taken in evaluating evidence to allow reliable conclusions than was the case in other disciplines. But the struggle with these difficulties has had a remarkable consequence. As the science became more and more important it began to have a greater and greater effect on the profession itself, so that medicine as a profession has become scientific to an extent that exceeds many others. The influential physician Archie Cochrane, whom we shall encounter again in Chapter 8, had this to say about the medical profession. 'What other profession encourages publications about its error, and experimental investigations into the effect of their actions? Which magistrate, judge or headmaster has encouraged RCTs [randomised clinical trials] into their 'therapeutic' and 'deterrent' actions?'[16]

In this book we shall look at the role that medical statistics has come to play in scientific medicine. We shall do this by looking not only at current evidential challenges but also at the history of the subject. This has two advantages. It leavens the statistical with the historical but it also gives a much fairer impression of the difficulties. The physicians and statisticians we shall encounter were explorers. In the famous story of Columbus's egg, the explorer, irritated at being told that his exploits were easy, challenged the guests at a banquet to balance an egg on its end. When all had failed, he succeeded by flattening one end by tapping it against the table, a trick that any would then have been able to repeat. Repetition is easier than innovation.

We shall not delay our quest any further and who better to start with than one who was not only a mathematician but also a physician. However, he was also much more than that: a notable translator, a man of letters and a wit. A Scot who gave the English one of their most enduring symbols, he was something of a paradox, but although this has been a chapter of paradoxes, we must proceed to the next one if we wish to understand his significance.

2

The diceman cometh

'I lisped in numbers, for the numbers came'[1]

Pope, *Epistle to Dr. Arbuthnot*

An epistle from Dr. Arbuthnot

We need to reclaim Dr. John Arbuthnot[2] from literature for statistics. I doubt that he would thank us for it. He was by all accounts a delightful man, a friend of Pope's and of Swift's, not only witty and hugely and variously talented but modest as well. It is reasonable to assume that he was popular with his contemporaries on the basis of his agreeable conversation in the coffee-house rather than for his skills as a calculator. Indeed, he is now chiefly remembered as a literary character rather than as a mathematical figure. Yet, his literary fame is of a peculiar kind. We remember him for something he did not write and have all but forgotten that his most lasting creation is by him. It is a safe bet that more people can name Pope's *Epistle to Dr. Arbuthnot* than any work by Dr. John himself and how many know that he is the creator of John Bull?

Arbuthnot was born in 1667 in the Scottish village of the same name that lies between Montrose and Stonehaven, a few miles inland from Inverbervie. He showed an early interest in mathematics and in 1692 translated into English the important treatise on probability, *De Ratiociniis in Ludo Aleae,* by Dutch astronomer Christiaan Huygens (1629–1695). He originally studied at Marischal College Aberdeen but graduated in 1696 from St Andrews with a medical degree.

Arbuthnot then went to London where he gave lessons in mathematics. He was soon practising medicine instead and in 1705 was appointed as a physician to Queen Anne. He was elected a Fellow of the Royal Society in 1704.[3] It is for a paper that he read to the Royal Society on 19 April 1711, 'An argument for divine providence taken from the constant regularity observ'd in the births of both sexes',[4] that he is of interest to statisticians.

Arbuthnot's paper is notable for two reasons. The first is that it represents an early application of probabilistic reasoning to data. Hitherto, as in the treatise by Huygens that Arbuthnot had translated, probability had been mainly applied to games of chance. Data had been used for statistical reasoning before Arbuthnot, of course. John Graunt and William Petty, in England, and Johann De Witt in the Netherlands had used vital statistics and even constructed life tables (a topic we shall encounter in Chapter 7), but these calculations made little direct use of the mathematics of probability. Arbuthnot was to apply probability directly to statistics that he had for christenings, year by year for 82 years from 1629–1710. The type of probability calculation that he performed is what we should now call a *significance test* and is one of the most common forms of statistical argument employed today. This constitutes the second feature of interest of his paper. John Arbuthnot has a good claim to be the father of the significance test.

Statistics of births and the birth of statistics

Arbuthnot had data on the numbers of christenings in London by sex of the child. The data are represented in Figure 2.1. This is a modern form of representation, a plot of a *time series*, that was unknown to Arbuthnot and was not developed until the work of William Playfair (1759–1823). What is noticeable from the data is, first, that the christenings show considerable variation from year to year,[5] second, that the general pattern for males and females is very similar but, third, that the females christened year by year are always fewer in number than the males. For one or two years this latter feature is not so obvious. However, Figure 2.2 showing the ratios of males christened to females christened year by year makes this clear. The value of this ratio is always greater than 1.

It was this third feature of the data, clear from a careful inspection of Arbuthnot's original table, which particularly impressed him. As he pointed out, males had a higher mortality than females, and it was therefore appropriate that more should be born in order that each should find a mate. He set about examining the question, 'could the excess of males have arisen by chance?' The general question, 'could some pattern in the data have arisen by chance?' is central to the significance test as it is applied today.

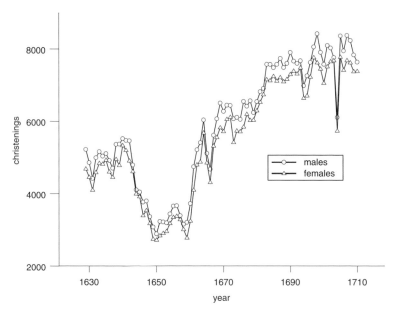

Figure 2.1 Time series plot of Arbuthnot's data.

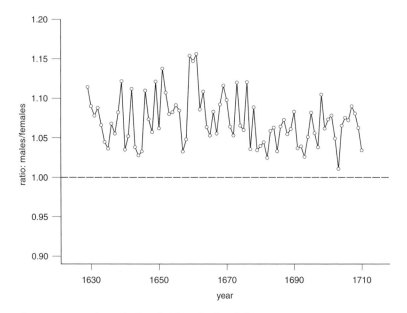

Figure 2.2 Sex ratio (males/females) for Arbuthnot's data.

Arbuthnot establishes what we should now refer to as a *null hypothesis* (a concept we encountered in Chapter 1). This is a hypothesis about some state of nature satisfying three conditions. First it is a hypothesis we are seeking to overturn, second it is a default hypothesis we shall consider 'true' unless disproved and third it is a hypothesis that defines the probabilities of some suitable statistic taking on given values. A helpful analogy is with Anglo-Saxon law. The scientist acts as prosecuting counsel and the null hypothesis is the presumed innocence of the defendant. (In making this analogy, I am not suggesting that the law *ought* to proceed along the lines of classical significance testing.)

In this case Arbuthnot's null hypothesis is that, if chance dictated all, the sex ratio at birth ought to be 1 rather than $^{14}/_{13}$, which is approximately the figure observed in his series. Arbuthnot does not discuss the possibility that the ratio for christenings might not reflect that for births. Instead he proceeds to investigate a question that is ancillary to his main purpose: 'if the probability of a male and that of a female birth are the same, what is the probability that we will see the same number of each?'

In order to illustrate this problem he considers the analogy of a two-sided die (a curious construction!) with faces marked M and F, 'which denote Cross and Pile'. Arguments involving such devices would be familiar to him as the translator of Huygens's work. First we may note that if we have an odd number of births then clearly we cannot have equal numbers of males and females. Arbuthnot points out that the probabilities of a given number of crosses and piles in n rolls of a die can be given by the binomial expansion of $(M + F)^n$ and uses this to consider the probability of equal numbers of males and females when the number of births is even. For example, if the die is rolled twice we have $(M + F)^2 = M^2 + 2MF + F^2$. If it is rolled four times we have $M^4 + 4M^3F + 6M^2F^2 + 4MF^3 + F^4$. The middle term in each of these two series is the case corresponding to equal numbers of each of M and F. Take the second of these series. The coefficient of each term in turn is 1, 4, 6, 4 and 1, making a total of 16. If M and F are equally likely, then the probability of each of these terms differs only according to the coefficient attached to it. Hence out of 16 cases in total, 6 correspond to exact equality and the probability we require is $^6/_{16}$. Table 2.1 illustrates all possible sequences of two rolls and four rolls of the die, grouping them in the way given by the binomial expansion to make clear what Arbuthnot is illustrating here.

Next, Arbuthnot considers the following situation: suppose that one man bet another that every year more males will be born than females,

Table 2.1. *A listing of all possible sequences for two and for four rolls of Arbuthnot's two-sided die.*

	Two trials		
M²	2MF	F²	
MM	MF	FF	
	FM		

		Four trials		
M⁴	4M³F	6M²F²	4MF³	F⁴
MMMM	MMMF	MMFF	MFFF	FFFF
	MMFM	MFMF	FMFF	
	MFMM	MFFM	FFMF	
	FMMM	FMMF	FFFM	
		FMFM		
		FFMM		

what is the 'value of his expectation?'. Arbuthnot's previous argument has shown that there are two different cases: that where the number of births is odd and that where it is even. In the former case, exact equality is impossible. That being so, either male births are in the excess, or females are. If 'the die' is fair, each of these two cases is equally likely. Therefore, the probability of a male excess is one-half. If, on the other hand, the number of births is even, the probability of males being in excess is less than one-half since there is also the possibility of an exact match.

Arbuthnot has thus established that the probability of an excess of male births in one year is less than or equal to one-half. The exact probability is rather difficult to manage in general and so Arbuthnot now uses a device to which statisticians still commonly resort when the exact handling of probabilities is delicate: he uses a conservative approximation. He proposes to use the value one-half in the rest of his calculations: either this value will be exactly true or it will be nearly true (given a large number of births) but slightly in excess of the true value.

Significant theology

Arbuthnot now calculates the probability that year in year out for 82 years, the male births will exceed the female births in number. Using his previously established probability of one-half, this probability is simply the product of one-half with itself 82 times, or $(1/2)^{82} = 1/2^{82}$. As we know from the story of the man who invented chess and bankrupted the maharaja who granted his request that he be given one grain of wheat for the first square, two grains for the second and so forth, the number of grains for the last square being 2^{63}, numbers grow fast by doubling. They also shrink fast by halving: $1/2^{82}$ is the reciprocal of a very large number indeed and hence represents a minute probability. Arbuthnot calculates this to be 1/4 836 000 000 000 000 000 000 000. There are 21 zeros in this and your chance of winning the UK national lottery *three weeks in a row* is more than a thousand times greater.[6]

Since Arbuthnot has given the 'null hypothesis' the benefit of the doubt by allowing the probability to be one-half in all years, when it must be slightly less in some, his minute probability is if anything too large. Arbuthnot concludes that consequently, 'it is Art, not Chance, that governs'.

We need not concern ourselves here with the reasonableness of Arbuthnot's conclusion, except to note that if the die is not fair in the first place but has a tendency to favour males, the result is not remarkable. In a sense, this is the *alternative hypothesis*, that Arbuthnot has established by rejecting his null. Tastes will differ as to whether this requires a theological explanation. However, there is a feature of Arbuthnot's test that requires further comment.

Suppose that he had arranged his observations on a weekly basis instead. In that case he would have averaged just over 113 males and 106 females for a series of approximately 4280 weeks. It is almost certain that in some of those weeks females would have exceeded males, the expected numbers 113 and 106 being too small to guarantee an excess amongst the observed cases. In fact, using the very same binomial distribution as Arbuthnot, but allowing that the probability of a male birth is 113/(113 + 106) = 113/219 = 0.516, it can be calculated that the probability of 109 or fewer male births for a total of 219 births, which implies that females are in the majority, is greater than 0.3. Thus about three-tenths of all the weeks would show an excess of female births.[7]

This raises two problems. The first is the rather arbitrary nature of the particular statistic used to investigate the null hypothesis: a regularity in years rather than decades, months, weeks or days. The second is that it points out the necessity of being able to calculate appropriate probabilities when the most extreme case has *not* been observed. As argued above, had Arbuthnot used weekly data he would have been faced with a situation in which about seven weeks in every ten would have shown an excess of male births. Over a long series of 4280 weeks this would have been a remarkable excess over what would be expected on an equal chance, but the fact that the excess was not extreme poses a particular problem. How does one conduct a significance test when the most extreme case has not arisen?

To answer that question, we shall turn to the case of Bernoulli.

Bernoulli numbers

Bernoulli[8] is a peculiar mathematician but not singular. On the contrary, he is plural and it is *this* that makes him peculiar. In fact he is a whole *tribe* of Swiss mathematicians. If we have difficulty in distinguishing Alexandre Dumas *père* from Alexandre Dumas *fils*, get confused about the Johann Bachs and have the odd spot of bother with the Pieter Breughels and others of that genre, this is nothing compared with our difficulties with the Bernoullis, who comprise, at least, three Johns, three Nicholases, two Daniels and two Jameses, not to mention a Christopher and a John-Gustave.[9] A partial family tree is shown in Figure 2.3.

The familial involvement in mathematics followed a familiar pattern. The father, who in most cases was himself one of the famous Bernoulli mathematicians, would resolutely oppose his son's interest in the subject, suggesting instead a career in business or one of the professions,

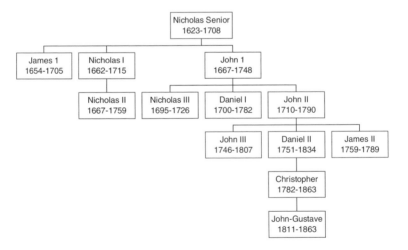

Figure 2.3 Family tree of the Bernoullis (based on Boyer[10]).

usually medicine or the Church. The son would duly take up some non-mathematical occupation but then, reverting to ancestral type, astonish the world with his mathematical brilliance and upset his father, by usurping his place in the mathematical pantheon, like some god in a Greek myth. In *Men of Mathematics*,[11] E. T. Bell takes this as being a clear demonstration of the importance of genetic inheritance in forming the intellect. The Bernoullis, however, were Protestants of Calvinist stock and may have seen it as a vindication of predestination.

The founder of this remarkable dynasty was Nicholas Bernoulli,[12] a drug merchant. Since he himself did not practise mathematics, he does not figure in the list of famous mathematicians. However, by the same token, he can also be absolved of all accusations of hypocrisy in advising sons to avoid dealing with any numbers that did not have a Franc attached to them. My own experience in drug development has taught me how sound his advice is. Marketing holds out greater prospects than statistics. The challenge of selling effective remedies to desperate patients who don't have to pay for them should never be overestimated. On the other hand, nothing is quite as satisfying as mathematics, and statistics, its homely cousin, shares a little in this glory.

A Daniel comes to judgement

Daniel I is the Bernoulli who interests us here. He was a very great mathematician but it is not quite right of me to have referred to him so far as 'Bernoulli' *tout court*. He is the greater of the two Daniels, so we can drop the I, but he is not undisputedly the greatest of the dozen or so Bernoullis, so that we cannot refer to him simply as Bernoulli. That claim, at least as far as statisticians are concerned, belongs to his uncle, James I (1654–1705), whose great work on probability, *Ars Conjectandi*, was published in 1713, eight years after his death. Mathematicians might dispute the claim that James was the greatest of the Bernoullis and assert his brother John claims instead. Physicists might advance the claims of Daniel. If Daniel is not the principal Bernoulli he is at least the author of 'The Bernoulli principle', the basis of heavier-than-air flight.

Daniel's father was James's younger brother John and, true to family tradition, he discouraged his son's interest in mathematics, decrying his talent and advising him to enter business. Instead Daniel studied medicine, but soon showed dangerous mathematical tendencies. His father relented and gave Daniel extra classes in mathematics. Daniel's medical dissertation, *De Respiratione*, was really about mechanics and described a new sort of spirometer. He later unwisely entered a competition for a prize in mathematics offered by the French Academy of Sciences. His father John then discovered that although the coveted prize had been awarded to 'Bernoulli' it was not to him alone, as he had at first supposed, and would have to be shared. Enraged, John then banned his presumptuous son from the house.

In the meantime, Daniel had contributed to the eastward expansion of the new mathematics (the Bernoullis were originally from Antwerp, where Daniel's great-grandparents had fled religious persecution to settle in Basle) by following his brother Nicholas, also a mathematician, to St. Petersburg. Daniel was later joined by his friend and fellow Basler Leonhard Euler (1707–1783). Daniel did not stay in Russia long, however. He returned to Basle and contributed to many fields of mathematics and physics whilst continuing to attract his father's ire. In fact, if the Belgian feminist philosopher Luce Irigaray's thesis on masculine and feminine physics,[13] so admirably discussed in Sokal and Bricmont's *Impostures Intellectuelles*,[14] is correct, not only were father and son eminent mathematicians, they must have been feminists before their time, since the next thing they disagreed about was fluid dynamics. Apparently, this is an example of 'feminine physics', being concerned with that which is soft and hence by definition feminine and which has consequently been sadly neglected by male physicists and mathematicians, with the exception, of course, of the Bernoullis, Newton, Euler, D'Alembert, Lagrange, Stokes, Navier and all the others. We may also note that if only the great 19th century female mathematician Sonja Kowalewski had had the benefit of a post-modernist and structuralist education she would have known that the mathematics of solid bodies is a male subject and would not have wasted her time writing the paper on this topic that won the Bordin Prize of the French Academy of Sciences.[15] To return to the Bernoullis, Daniel published a masterly work on this subject (fluid dynamics), *Hydrodynamica*, in 1738. John published a work entitled *Hydrolica* on the same subject, in the same year, faking an earlier publication date, and each claimed the other was a plagiarist.

From significant stars to stars for significance

However, this is not the reason we are interested in Daniel here. That has to do instead with a treatise of his on astronomy, which includes a section applying probability to the problem of planetary orbits. The ecliptic is the plane of the Earth as it journeys around the Sun. The other planets have orbits whose planes are closely aligned to the ecliptic, with the possible exception of Pluto, whose angle of inclination is 17°. However, Pluto was undiscovered in Daniel's day as was Neptune. Uranus was discovered by Herschel in 1781, the year before Daniel's death, but this was long after Daniel's treatise, which dates from 1734 and is yet another prize-winner in the Paris competition.

The inclinations of the orbits of the planets known to Daniel are as follows,[16]

Mercury	7.0°
Venus	3.4°
Mars	1.9°
Jupiter	1.3°
Saturn	2.5°

from which we may discover that if men are from Mars and women are from Venus, eccentrics come from Mercury, which at 7° has the largest angle. Since the maximum possible angle a planet's orbit could have to the ecliptic would be 90°, this pattern is obviously far from 'random'. The question that Daniel sought to answer was, 'can we prove it is not random?'.[17]

In fact, Daniel seeks to answer this in a number of ways.[18] For example, he actually considers the difference between all pairs of planetary orbits (not just taking the Earth as the reference point) and discovers that the biggest difference is between the Earth and Mercury. The solution to this problem is too difficult for us to consider here. However, he also compares all the planetary orbits to the Sun's own equator obtaining the following results:

Mercury	2°56′
Venus	4°10′
Earth	7°30′
Mars	5°49′
Jupiter	6°21′
Saturn	5°58′

Here we have the Earth's orbit as providing the most extreme value. We shall consider Daniel's analysis of these data. This problem raises rather different issues from Arbuthnot's. To see why, return to Arbuthnot's example and suppose (ignoring the problem with weekly series of christenings) that we postulate an alternative hypothesis: 'divine providence will always intervene to ensure that in a given year, more males than females will be born'. What is the probability of the observed data under this hypothesis? The answer is clearly 1 and this means that Arbuthnot's probability of $(1/2)^{82}$ is not only the probability of the observed event given that the null hypothesis is true, it is also the *ratio* of that probability to the probability of the observed event under the alternative hypothesis.

Probabilities of events (or the collection of events we record in data sets) given hypotheses are called *likelihood*, by statisticians, which is used by them to have this technical meaning only. The concept and term are due the great British statistician and geneticist R. A. Fisher (1890–1962), as we explained in the last chapter. Arbuthnot's probability can also be interpreted as a ratio of likelihoods. Such ratios are commonly used by statisticians to express the extent to which the data support one hypothesis compared to the other.

But now suppose that we try and apply this concept to Daniel Bernoulli's question. We immediately have a difficulty. If our alternative hypothesis is, 'the planetary orbits have been arranged to be perfectly coplanar with the sun's equator', then this produces a likelihood of zero, since the data flatly contradict *this* hypothesis. The ratio of likelihoods in favour of the 'distributed at random' hypothesis is thus infinite (or *undefined*, to be mathematically nice). However, our intuition tells us that this random hypothesis is incompatible with the observed results. Perhaps we should consider an alternative 'alternative', namely, 'the planetary orbits have been arranged to be *nearly* coplanar'. The problem with this is that it is too vague and will not allow us to calculate a probability.

Perhaps we can return to our first interpretation of Arbuthnot's calculation: as a probability under the null hypothesis with no reference to the alternative. We can try to apply this to Daniel Bernoulli's problem. Suppose, in fact, that we can only measure the angles to the nearest degree. We could then argue that any value between 1 and 90 is equally likely. There being five planets, the probability of the results exactly observed is thus $(1/90)^5$, a gratifyingly small value. There is, however, something obviously inappropriate about this. Whatever the results had been, by calculating in this particular way, we would always obtain a value of $(1/90)^5$, since under the null hypothesis of random distribution, each angle is equally likely.

An alternative argument then forms the basis of the significance test and goes something like this.

> Q. What feature of the data particularly strikes us?
>
> A. The fact that the largest angle is equal to $7°30'$.
>
> Q. Would we not find it even more striking if the maximum angle were $6°$?
>
> A. Of course. And it would be even more striking if it were $5°$, and yet more striking if it were $4°$ and so forth.
>
> Q. In that case, what is the probability of *any* of these cases?
>
> A. That is the probability that the maximum angle is *less than or equal* to $7°30'$.

Assuming that all angles are equally likely the probability that any given angle is less than or equal to $7°30' = 7°30'/90° = 1/12$. Hence the probability that they are all less than $7°30'$ if distributed randomly is $1/12^6 = 1/12\,985\,984$. This is, in fact, the figure that Daniel obtains. Nowadays we would regard this result as 'highly significant' and award it several stars.

The smallness of this probability is then taken as being an indication of the degree to which the data (fail to) support the null hypothesis. Such a probability, the probability of observing a result as extreme *or more extreme*[19] than the result observed is what statisticians call a 'P-value'. Both Arbuthnot's and Daniel Bernoulli's probabilities can be regarded as P-values. In Arbuthnot's case however, the 'more extreme' part is irrelevant since he has the most extreme result.

Modern significance tests are particularly associated with R. A. Fisher (see below), who contributed considerably to their development, and have the following features.

1. We establish a null hypothesis.
2. We choose a statistic (e.g. the largest angle of inclination).
3. The null hypothesis defines the probability distribution of that statistic.
4. We have a means of defining what constitutes more extreme values of this statistic.
5. We calculate the probability of observing a result as extreme or more extreme than that observed.

This probability is then either reported as a P-value or compared to some probabilistic yardstick, most typically 5%. In the latter case a decision is made to reject (the probability is less than or equal to the yardstick) or not reject (the probability is greater that the yardstick) the null hypothesis. Usually it is considered important to have defined steps 1, 2 and 4 in advance of examining the data. This is possible in the context of drug development, for example, but not in many other cases and not, in particular, in those considered by Arbuthnot and Bernoulli.

The Reverend Bayes and his irreverent followers

'Life', the statistician Maurice Kendal once remarked, 'would be much simpler if the Bayesians followed the example of their master and published posthumously'. He was referring to the fact that the chief claim to fame of Thomas Bayes (1701–1761) is a work, entitled, *An Essay Towards Solving a Problem in the Doctrine of Chance* and communicated to the Royal Society in 1763 by his friend Richard Price.

The place of Thomas Bayes's birth is a subject fit for Bayesian speculation. Some bet on London and others Hertfordshire.[20] It has been discovered only relatively recently that he studied theology in Edinburgh.[21] In 1694, his father Joshua was the first non-conformist minister to be ordained publicly after the act of Uniformity was passed.[22] He became a minister at Leather Lane in London in 1723 and Thomas served as his assistant. By 1731, Thomas was himself a Presbyterian minister in Tunbridge Wells. As regards the flame of scientific fame, Bayes is a slow burner. Although elected as Fellow of the Royal Society in 1742, there is no evidence of his ever having published during his lifetime any work of mathematics under his own name. He was originally omitted from the *Dictionary of National Biography* and when R. A. Fisher wrote to the editors trying to get him included: he was informed that such errors of omission were not rectified.[23] He would have completely disappeared from our historical consciousness but for the posthumous publication arranged by his friend Price.

Thomas Bayes would be astonished at his scientific afterlife. There is a large and vigorous movement 'Bayesian statistics' named after him. Every year hundreds if not thousands of scientific articles are published using the adjective Bayesian in their titles. The Bayesians themselves meet every four years in Valencia (or nearby[24]) where, in addition to presenting each other papers on their favourite topic, they have social evenings in which they all join in singing anthems such as, *There's no Business like Bayes Business*, *Bayesian Boy*, *Bayesians in the Night* ('Something in your prior \ was so exciting \ Something in your data \ was so inviting . . .') and other ditties of mind-numbing puerility.

However, if Bayesians at play are a nauseating sight, Bayesians at work are most impressive and the Bayesian *œuvre* as a whole is a magnificent contribution to the philosophy of knowledge. In order to explain exactly what they are up to, it will be necessary to take a slight diversion to cover more fully a matter we touched on briefly in Chapter 1: the difference between probability and statistics.

This book is about the contribution that the science of statistics has made and is making to the life sciences, in particular medicine. It is not directly concerned with the subject of probability, which is really a branch of mathematics. This may seem rather surprising, as the statistician appears to be continually involved in the business of calculating probabilities. The difference is really the difference between the divine and the human. Probability is a divine subject, whereas statistics is human.

What I mean by this is that probability, unlike statistics, needs no starting point in experience. Indeed, many do not consider that the subject was fully developed until axiomised in 1933 by the great Russian mathematician A. N. Kolmogorov (1903–1987).[25] Nowadays any serious treatment of probability will start with the axioms and proceed to working out the consequences. To the extent that they ever actually involve numbers, the numerical problems always begin with a 'given'. 'Given that we have a fair coin, what is the probability of obtaining six heads in ten tosses?' is an example of the species, albeit far too simple to be interesting to a probabilist. The point about the 'given' is that it is never found. It must always be supplied. In practice, it could only ever be supplied by the Almighty. Hence the divine or religious nature of probability. A probability argument starts with a fiat: 'let there be theta'.[26]

Statistics on the other hand is human. It deals with the reverse problem. It treats the data as known and the probability as to be found. It answers problems of this sort, '*Given* the number of times in which an unknown event has happened and failed: *Required* the chance that the probability of its happening in a single trial lies somewhere between any two degrees of probability that that can be named.' The quotation is from Bayes's famous essay. Statistics needs mathematics to answer this question but cannot rely on mathematics alone. It is thus, from the mathematician's point of view, a far dirtier and less respectable subject than probability. Thus, to put it simply, probability is the business of arguing from presumed model to potential data whereas statistics is the business of inferring models from known data. It deals with what has come to be known as 'the problem of inverse probability'.

The various schools of statistics deal with this in different ways. The majority frequentist approach is to postpone the moment at which the

Table 2.2. *An example from screening to illustrate Bayes theorem.*

Status	Sign		Total
	−	+	
Well	800	100	900
Ill	25	75	100
Total	825	175	1000

divine becomes human as long as possible (the method of the awaited avatar). An attempt is made to continue in the general framework of probability as long as possible. The significance tests of Arbuthnot and Daniel Bernoulli illustrate this approach. It is assumed that a particular state of nature applies. A contingent probability calculation follows. This contingent calculation appears to be able to proceed objectively. Only at the very end is the business of judging whether the hypothesis is reasonable attempted.

The Bayesian approach is different. The calculation requires as initial input a probability that the hypothesis is true (the approach of the immediate incarnation). It thus starts with what is usually referred to as a *prior probability*. But this probability has, of necessity, to be subjective. This subjective prior is then combined with the likelihood (the probability of the data given a hypothesis) to form a posterior distribution, using *Bayes theorem*, the posthumous contribution of Thomas Bayes to statistics.

Screen test*

Bayes's original argument is too technical for us to follow here. Instead, to illustrate 'Bayes theorem', we shall consider a simple (fictitious) example from screening. Consider a small closed population consisting of 1000 individuals. Suppose that we can classify these individuals as either well or ill and also according to the presence or absence of some 'sign' as positive or negative. Table 2.2 represents the situation.

We shall now use this table to define three kinds of probability: *joint, marginal* and *conditional*. Suppose that we select an individual at random from the population, what is the probability that this individual will be ill with a positive sign? This is an example of a *joint* probability since it involves the joint occurrence of two events: ill and positive. There are 75 such individuals out of a total population of 1000 so that the required probability is $75/1000 = 0.075$.

Now consider instead an example of a *marginal* probability. What is the probability that an individual chosen at random is ill? This probability can be obtained by using the marginal total of ill patients, which is 100, and dividing it by the overall number of 1000. We thus have a probability of $100/1000 = 0.1$. Note also that the marginal probability is the sum of joint probabilities. It is the sum of the joint probability of being 'positive' and ill, which we have already seen is 0.075, and of being 'negative' and ill which may be seen to be 0.025.

Finally consider a conditional probability: the probability that an individual chosen at random is 'positive' given that the individual is ill. There are 100 ill individuals, 75 of whom are positive so that the requisite probability is $75/100 = 0.75$.

Now, note that the joint probability can be expressed as the product of a marginal probability and a conditional probability: $0.075 = 0.1 \times 0.75$. This is, in fact, a general rule of probability and may be expressed thus. Given two events A & B, the joint probability of their occurrence is the product of the marginal probability of A and the conditional probability of B given A. Symbolically we have $P(A \cap B) = P(A)P(B \mid A)$. The so-called intersection symbol $\cap$ is used to denote 'and' and the vertical division $\mid$ to denote 'given', with brackets signifying 'of' and P standing for probability. However, it turns out that this formula can equally well be expressed in terms of marginal probabilities of B and conditional probabilities of A as $P(A \cap B) = P(B)P(A \mid B)$. For example, the marginal probability that an individual is positive is $175/1000 = 0.175$ and the probability that the individual is ill given that the individual is positive is $75/175 = 3/7$. The product of the two is $0.175 \times 3/7 = 0.075$ as before.

It is worth stressing, as an aside at this point, that to assume that the probability of A given B is the same as that of B given A is to make an egregious error in logic, of the sort one does not expect to encounter, except daily in the news media and our courts of law. It is comparable to assuming that '"I see what I eat" is the same thing as "I eat what I see"', a point of view that you would have to be madder than a March Hare to hold.[27] We can illustrate this with our example. Most ill members of the population are positive, and the conditional probability of the latter in the population defined by the former is 0.75. However, it does not follow that most positive people are ill and, indeed, the requisite probability is only $3/7$. To give another more forceful example, most women do not die of breast cancer; however, the overwhelming majority of breast cancer deaths are to women.

Returning to our examination of probabilities, we may thus also write $P(B \cap A) = P(B)P(AB)$. It therefore follows that we can equate the two right-hand sides of these equations to obtain,

$$P(B)P(A \mid B) = P(A)P(B \mid A)$$

from which, dividing through by $P(B)$ we have,

$$P(A \mid B) = P(A)P(B \mid A)/P(B)$$

This is Bayes theorem.

To see the utility of this theorem to a system of statistical inference, consider that we wish to discover the probability of a particular hypothesis given some data. If we have H standing for hypothesis and D standing for data, we can then, substituting H for A and D for B, re-write Bayes theorem as:

$$P(H \mid D) = P(H)P(D \mid H)/P(D)$$

A linguistic statement to parallel this algebraic one would be as follows. 'The probability of a hypothesis given some data that has been observed is equal to the probability of the hypothesis multiplied by the probability of the data given the hypothesis and divided by the probability of the data.' One begins to appreciate the value of symbols! Whether expressed in words or symbols, Bayes theorem would thus appear to give us a means of calculating the probability of a hypothesis given the data.

However, in practice there are two formidable difficulties. The first is to do with the term $P(H)$. This is the marginal probability of the hypothesis. Which is to say it is the probability of the hypothesis without specifying any particular data. In other words, it is the probability of the hypothesis in ignorance of the data. Hence it can be regarded as a *prior* probability: the probability that would apply to the hypothesis before data have been collected. The second difficulty is the term $P(D)$. This is the marginal probability of the data. That is to say it is the probability of the data without specifying any particular hypothesis. It is thus a form of marginal probability. As we have already seen, a marginal probability can be obtained as the sum of relevant joint probabilities. The relevant joint probabilities in this case are those applying *to all possible hypotheses* and the data observed. If these are summed over all possible hypotheses, we obtain the marginal probability of the data. These hypotheses, let alone their joint probability with the data, are often extremely difficult to establish. The reader who doubts this might like to have a go at Daniel Bernoulli's problem.

If, however, we are just interested in the relative probability of two hypotheses, the second of the two difficulties in applying Bayesian thinking can be finessed. Suppose that we have two hypotheses, let us call them H_A, and H_B, for both of which we can establish probabilities of the data observed. (Recall that such probabilities are referred to as likelihoods.) By Bayes theorem we have

$$P(H_A \mid D) = P(H_A)P(D \mid H_A)/P(D) \text{ and also}$$
$$P(H_B \mid D) = P(H_B)P(D \mid H_B)/P(D),$$

the most difficult term in each expression being $P(D)$. Suppose, however, that we are interested in the ratios of the probabilities (the 'odds') on the left-hand side of each expression. We can express these as the ratio of the terms on the right-hand side. The common term $P(D)$ cancels out and we are left with

$$\frac{P(H_A \mid D)}{P(H_B \mid D)} = \frac{P(H_A)}{P(H_B)} \times \frac{P(D \mid H_A)}{P(D \mid H_B)}.$$

The ratio on the left-hand side of this expression is the *posterior odds* of hypothesis A relative to B. (How many times more probable A is compared to B as a result of seeing the data we have obtained.) The first term on the right-hand side is the *prior odds*. The second term on the right-hand side is the ratio of likelihoods that we already encountered in our discussion of Arbuthnot. Thus, in this form, Bayes theorem becomes:

posterior odds = prior odds × ratio of likelihoods.

Of the two terms on the right, the second is, in a sense, objective. It is the ratio of two likelihoods, each of which is established as a more or less formal consequence of the hypothesis in question. This may, of course, involve some complex calculation but the result is at least to some degree inherent in the problem rather than a function of the calculator's beliefs. The first term, however, must be produced from thin air. It represents belief. It is this in particular that makes Bayesian statistics controversial.

Laplace transforms probability

As we have seen, a principal objection to the use of Bayesian methods concerns prior distributions. Schematically the Bayesian argument can be represented as:

Prior Opinion + Likelihood → Posterior Opinion.

Since likelihood is the mathematical embodiment of the data, its probabilistic essence, it is hard to see what is objectionable in this. We have opinions, we make observations, we change our opinions. This is surely a description of the way that humans think (bigots excepted, of course!).

However, scientists are uncomfortable with the subjective. The most important of Bayes's immediate successors, Simon Pierre de Laplace, was to promote an influential way of banishing the subjective,[28] or at least appearing to do so. We divert briefly to consider his career.

Unlike Bayes, Laplace (1749–1827)[29] is a major mathematician whose importance far exceeds his contribution to statistics. In addition to his work on probability theory, he is principally remembered for his contributions to the solutions of differential equations and also to celestial mechanics. As regards the latter he famously proved the stability of the solar system, which proof, in the light of modern chaos theory, no one takes seriously any more. However, Carlyle may have had Laplace in mind in *Sartor Resartus*: 'Is there no God then; but at best an absentee God, sitting idle, ever since the first Sabbath, at the outside of his Universe, and seeing it go?'[30]

On the personal and social level Laplace amply demonstrated the Bayesian necessity of maintaining enough flexibility in one's prior to permit judicious updating in the light of emerging evidence. He lived through several political changes in France, monarchy, revolution, directory, empire and back to monarchy, and prospered through all of them. He was made a member of the Academy before the revolution and was briefly Minister of the Interior under Napoleon. Napoleon dismissed him, joking that he, 'carried the spirit of the infinitely small into the management of affairs'[31] but he also awarded Laplace the Grand Cross of the Legion of Honour, the Order of the Réunion and made him a Count of the Empire. Laplace repaid these honours by being a signatory to the order that banished Bonaparte, and Louis XVIII made him a marquis.[32]

Laplace had another rather unpleasant habit that we have already encountered with some of the Bernoullis. He was not always careful to give priority. Opinion is thus divided as to whether or not he discovered Bayes theorem independently in 1774 some ten years after Bayes's posthumous paper. It is quite possible that he is guiltless of plagiarism in this, as it may be that the French mathematicians were not conversant with Bayes's essay.[33]

'If an urn contains an infinite number of white and black tickets in unknown proportion and we draw $p + q$ tickets of which p are white and q are black; one requires the probability that in drawing a new ticket from this urn it will be white'.[34] Thus writes Laplace in his *Theorie analytique de probabilités*. In modern terms, Laplace seeks to estimate an unknown probability, θ, on the basis of data obtained to date. There are at least two ways in which we would now think of this unknown probability. One is as a *parameter*, the unknown proportion of tickets in the urn, the other is more directly as the probability that applies to the next ticket to be drawn. This latter is what is known to modern Bayesians as a *predictive probability* and appears to be closer to Laplace's intention. In this particular example it turns out that an appropriate *estimate* of the unknown parameter is the same as the predictive probability.

Laplace's solution is that the required probability is $(p + 1)/(p + q + 2)$. It can be seen that if no tickets have yet been drawn so that $p = q = 0$, the required probability is $1/2$. One way of looking at this formula is as follows. Imagine that as you draw your tickets you are going to build up your white and black tickets in two piles. To start the whole thing going before you draw any tickets you contribute one of appropriate colour to each pile. At any stage, your estimate as to the probability that the next one will be white is then the ratio of white tickets, including the one you originally contributed, to all tickets, including the two you originally contributed.

It may seem that this formula of Laplace's is absurd. Consider, for example, that we start out with the probability of one-half that the first ticket will be white. We also know in advance that having drawn one ticket our next estimate must either be $2/3$ if the ticket drawn was white or $1/3$ if it was black. But surely the true proportion of white tickets in the urn could be anything at all. Is it not ridiculous that we are limited to only two possible answers? Not necessarily. We are in danger of confusing an unknown probability with an estimate of that probability. Return to the position before any tickets are drawn. Suppose we now allow that the proportion of white tickets in the urn could be anything at all between 0 and 1. If we regard all of these values as equally likely, our average of these probabilities is simply $1/2$. Thus in saying that the proportion of white tickets in the urn is $1/2$ we are not saying that it is definitely $1/2$ but simply that this is our average feeling about the value and hence our best bet as to the true probability.

But what entitles us to regard all the probabilities as equally likely? This is Laplace's famous (or infamous) *principle of insufficient reason*. 'When one has no *a priori* information of an event, one must consider all possibilities, from zero to one, equally likely'.[35] Unfortunately, in general, there is insufficient reason for the principle of insufficient reason. Consider the example of tossing a coin. Having tossed it once and having seen it come up heads would you regard the probability of its showing a head a second time as being $^2/_3$? Most people would want a value closer to $^1/_2$. This is because they would not regard each value between 0 and 1 as being equally likely in the first place. Of course, one could argue that this is because we have *a priori* information, if not on this coin then on the tossing of similar coins. But this is simply to admit that the principle of insufficient reason will rarely apply to anything and leaves us with the problem of what to use instead.

To cut a long story short

In Frederick C. Crews's wonderful pastiche anthology of literary criticism, *The Pooh Perplex*,[36] Murphy A. Sweat summarises 'Tom Mann's' *Magic Mountain* thus. 'It's about this bunch of birds who sit around an old health resort wondering if they're going to croak. Some do, some don't and then the book is over.' In what follows, we shall attempt an equivalent compression of some developments since Laplace.

As we have already mentioned, modern statistics is split between two major schools, the frequentist (sometimes referred to as classical) and the Bayesian or more properly the neo-Bayesian. A third school, the likelihood school, has a position that has some features of both schools. The reason that we should more properly refer to neo-Bayesian rather than Bayesian statistics is that when Bayesian methods re-emerged from the long dark winter to which R. A. Fisher's advances in statistics had condemned them, a radical shift in emphasis accompanied their use.

Ronald Aylmer Fisher was born on 17 February 1890, one of two twins, the other stillborn.[37] His early interest was in biology but he later claimed that it was the sight of a codfish skull and its labelled bones in a museum that dissuaded him from taking up a subject that seemed to involve rote memorisation.[38] Instead he elected to study mathematics and graduated from Cambridge as a wrangler in 1912,[39] staying on for a further year of postgraduate work in statistical mechanics, quantum theory and the theory of errors. He was, however, to retain his interest in biology all his life, in particular genetics and evolution, and the chairs that he held at

University College London (UCL), Cambridge and Adelaide were in genetics rather than statistics. He was also an enthusiastic member of the Eugenics Education Society of London.

Fisher has been described by Richard Dawkins as the greatest of Darwin's successors[40] and shares with J. B. S. Haldane, also of UCL, and the American Sewall Wright, the credit for reconciling Mendelian genetics and Darwinian evolution. However, he was an even greater statistician contributing to many theoretical and applied fields. He was the first to fully elucidate the concept of likelihood, made extensive contributions to the theory of estimation and significance testing, coined and developed analysis of variance and founded multivariate analysis.

He was also an opponent of Bayesian thinking. Fisher fell out early in his career with the leading statistician of the day (until Fisher supplanted him) Karl Pearson (1857–1936) Professor of Applied Mathematics and later Eugenics at UCL.[41] Pearson was a Bayesian and this may have influenced Fisher against that theory. Later, by which time Fisher himself was momentarily eclipsed by the Pole Jerzy Neyman[42] (1894–1981), who had developed an even more extreme alternative to Bayesian statistics during his time at UCL, Fisher's position on Bayesian approaches mellowed.

At the time that Fisher was developing his theories of statistical inference, the general mechanism that Laplace had bequeathed was still being employed in statistics. Many other fields had been opened up, in particular Francis Galton's discovery of correlation was being vigorously exploited by Karl Pearson and his colleagues, but the principle of insufficient reason together with Bayes theorem was what was being employed to generate statistical inferences.

An example can be given by considering Student's famous paper, On the Probable Error of a Mean.[43] Student (1876–1937), whose real name was William Sealy Gosset was an employee of the Guinness Company in Dublin and obtained leave to study with Karl Pearson at UCL.[44] (All the characters in this drama were at UCL at one time or another.) Student's practical work led him to make statistical inferences based on small samples but the methods then being used by Karl Pearson required large samples. How large is a large sample? How long is a piece of string? In fact until Student's work we didn't really know how large 'large' was. Nowadays we might place it at about 60 observations but possibly even as low as 20. Karl Pearson would have used 150 observations or so at least in his approaches.

Student did not illustrate the method he developed using data from his work as a brewer but from an early clinical trial which had been run at the Insane Asylum in Kalamazoo Michigan and organised by Arthur

Table 2.3. *The cushny and Peebles data (as quoted by Fisher quoting Student).*

Patient	A	B	Difference (B–A)
1	+0.7	+1.9	+1.2
2	−1.6	+0.8	+2.4
3	−0.2	+1.1	+1.3
4	−1.2	+0.1	+1.3
5	−0.1	−0.1	0.0
6	+3.4	+4.4	+1.0
7	+3.7	+5.5	+1.8
8	+0.8	+1.6	+0.8
9	0.0	+4.6	+4.6
10	+2.0	+3.4	+1.4
Mean	+7.5	+2.33	+1.58

Cushny, then professor at Michigan (later at UCL, of course) and his student Alvin Peebles.[45] Some of these data are reproduced in Table 2.3, as subsequently presented by R. A. Fisher[46] and represent the average hours of sleep gained by the use of two drugs for ten patients.

The effect of the drugs is measured with respect to a common baseline period and interest centres on the difference between the two which is given in the last column. This appears to suggest that B is the more effective hypnotic since, with the exception of patient number 5, for which there is no difference, the difference is always positive. The question naturally arises however, 'is this effect genuine or simply due to chance?' This question could in fact be answered using the method of John Arbuthnot. We could argue that under the null hypothesis of no difference, a positive or a negative difference is equally likely. If we then exclude those patients that show no difference then the probability of a positive difference on any patient that remains is $1/2$. There are nine such patients, patient 5 being excluded and so the probability we require is $(1/2)^9 = 1/512$. In the logic of the significance test we now have a fairly small probability and we either accept that an unusual event has occurred or reject the null hypothesis. We could also use Laplace's approach, setting $p = 9$ and $q = 1$, and estimate that the probability that a new patient, for whom a difference in hours sleep was obtained, would show a better effect with drug B. This would be $(9 + 1)/(9 + 1 + 2) = 10/12 = 0.83$.

In fact, Student does not reduce the data to signs only (positive or negative) but makes use of their magnitude also. The details of his calculations will not be covered but one aspect of them is worth noting. His object is to produce directly a Bayesian probability that B is better than A. Karl Pearson could have done this using 200 patients. Student's innovation consists in finding a method to do it for ten but this is not what interests us here. Both Pearson and Student would have agreed that the purpose of the calculation was to deliver directly a probability that B was better than A. Student calculates this probability to be 0.9985. Equivalently we can regard the probability that A is better than B as being $1 - 0.9985 = 0.0015$.

Implicitly Student's result relies on Bayes theorem together with an assumption of insufficient reason, that any possible true difference between the drugs is equally likely *a priori*. Indeed, this particular Bayesian approach to estimation was later extensively developed by the Cambridge astronomer Harold Jeffreys[47] (1891–1989). It is, however, what Fisher made of Student's paper that interests us. Fisher recognised the importance of Student's innovation in using small samples but gave the resulting probability a completely different interpretation. He pointed out that the probability of 0.0015 is not only the probability of A being superior to B given the joint use of Bayes theorem and the principle of insufficient reason, but that it is also the probability of observing a result as extreme or more extreme than that observed given that there is no difference between the drugs. This is, in fact, the *P*-value that we have encountered already in this chapter. Its calculation does not require a prior probability.

Although previous authors, notably Karl Pearson,[48] had given 'tail area' probabilities this *P*-value interpretation, it was Fisher who stressed this approach at the expense of others. Fisher popularised Student's test of 1908 and also his own interpretation of it in his influential book, *Statistical Methods for Research Workers* (1925) that eventually ran to 14 editions. His influence, together with a growing realisation that the principle of insufficient reason was unsatisfactory or at the very least impractical and the attractions of what appeared to be an objective alternative, may explain why Bayesian statistics went into a sharp decline from which it did not start to recover until the late 1950s. The ongoing story of that decline and its recovery, however, must wait until Chapter 4. Instead we now divert to have a look at one of the most important and controversial devices of the medical statistician, the clinical trial.

3

Trials of life

Everybody knows that the dice are loaded
Everybody rolls with their fingers crossed

Leonard Cohen

TB or notTB?

On 28 October 1948 a paper describing the outcome of the Medical Research Council trial of streptomycin in tuberculosis (TB) appeared in the *British Medical Journal*. The results were striking. Out of 55 patient treated with streptomycin only four died. On the other hand, of 52 control patients 14 died. Looked at in terms of patients who showed 'considerable improvement' the results were even more impressive: 28 in the streptomycin group and only 4 in the control group. Streptomycin had been shown to be an effective remedy against one of mankind's biggest killers and was, in due course, enrolled in the fight against the disease.

However, it is not for its successful conclusion that this trial is now chiefly remembered but for various innovations in design, including the application of *randomisation*. This trial is regarded as the first modern randomised clinical trial (RCT). As the paper put it, 'Determination of whether a patient would be treated by streptomycin and bed-rest (S case) or by bed-rest alone (C case) was made by reference to a statistical series based on random sampling numbers drawn up for each sex at each centre by Professor Bradford Hill; the details of the series were unknown to any of the investigators or to the co-ordinator and were contained in a set of sealed envelopes, each bearing on the outside only the name of the hospital and a number.'

Medecin manqué

Austin Bradford Hill (1897–1991) was born in Hampstead London, the son of Sir Leonard Erskine Hill, FRS, a famous physiologist.[1] A family legend had it that the Hills had given thought only to girls' names and were unprepared for the arrival of a boy. (Had they not read their Arbuthnot?) An alphabetical search for a boy's name got no further than Austin, a name that was never used anyway. The boy was always called Tony and the later added use of Bradford was to avoid confusion with the famous physiologist A. V. Hill.[2]

Bradford Hill contracted pulmonary TB when serving with the Royal Naval Air Service in the Aegean during the First World War. The streptomycin trial can be regarded as his revenge on the disease that thwarted his intention to pursue a medical career. He took a London University correspondence degree in economics instead. However, he was still interested in medicine and in 1922 he started work for the Industrial Fatigue Research Board. He worked with Major Greenwood[3] at the Medical Research Council Laboratories in Hampstead, but also attended Karl Pearson's lectures at University College London and gained a PhD for a dietary study.[4] Greenwood was appointed to the new Chair of Epidemiology and Vital Statistics at the London School of Hygiene and Tropical Medicine in 1927 and Bradford Hill moved with him. In 1933, Hill was appointed a reader and succeeded Greenwood as professor when he retired in 1945. He was made an FRS in 1954 and was knighted in 1961.

Bradford Hill was an extremely influential medical statistician but slightly unusual in some ways. Many who appear in this book had a foot in both camps: medicine and statistics. But in most cases, Daniel Bernoulli is a good example, it seems clear that their daemon drives them towards mathematics and away from medicine and this is, indeed, the way their careers move. Arbuthnot is, perhaps, an exception. Hill seems to have been another. He was always extremely interested in the medical applications of statistics and always took a special care to make his lectures clear and entertaining to a medical audience. A series of papers on statistics which he wrote for *The Lancet* were collected together in a book, which was published in 1937, and which ran to 11 editions in his lifetime.[5] He was famous for his wit and iconoclastic manner and was a superb after-dinner speaker. Despite his early brush with disease, Hill lived to enjoy a retirement of 30 years and did not die until 1991.

Square roots and diced vegetables

Hill would have been familiar with the idea of randomly allocating treatments from another context: the work of R. A. Fisher in the design of agricultural experiments. Graduating in 1912, Fisher stayed on at Cambridge for further postgraduate study in statistical mechanics, quantum theory and the theory of errors.[6] After leaving Cambridge in 1913 Fisher drifted through half a dozen jobs in as many years[7]: first in the City and then as a teacher of mathematics and physics at Rugby, Halibury, HM Training Ship Worcester and at Bradfield College. (His poor eyesight prevented his enlisting in the war.) He found the experience of teaching miserable and contemplated setting up as a subsistence farmer. However, in October 1919, aged 29, he joined the agricultural research station at Rothamsted in Harpenden as its first statistician and there began for him a remarkable period of fertile development of his statistical ideas. However, Fisher did not abandon his personal farming interests completely while at Rothamsted. He kept a goat, for example, and used to tether it on Harpenden Common on his way to work!

During the 14 years he stayed at Rothamsted,[8] he not only carried out the practical statistical investigations for which he had been hired, worked extensively on the theory of statistics and continued his researches in evolutionary genetics but also had the temerity to interfere in the design of the experiments being carried out by his colleagues. This irritating habit is, above all others, the hallmark of the modern statistician. As M. G. Kendall put it in *Hiawatha Designs an Experiment*, Hiawatha, who at college/Majored in applied statistics/Consequently felt entitled/To instruct his fellow man/In any subject whatsoever.

It had become the practice to run experiments with concurrent controls rather than by making historical comparisons. That is to say it was the practice to establish, for example, the effect of the application of a fertiliser on the yield of a crop by comparison to plots in the same field planted at the same time but to which no fertiliser had been applied. Fisher had good reason to know how important this was. One of his first tasks at Rothamsted had been to investigate the effect of the weather on the yield of 13 plots of the 'Broadbalk' wheat field that had had roughly uniform treatment from 1852 until 1918. Fisher was able to discern a number of factors affecting yield but puzzling peaks in the late 1850s and during the 1890s remained. He identified these periods as ones in which particular efforts had been made to weed the plots by hand. This sort of factor could very easily be overlooked and would bias conclusions if different years were compared with each other.

In deciding to assign treatments to various plots in a field, various restrictions might be observed. For example, it might be known that there was a fertility gradient in the field. One way of dealing with this was to allocate the treatments in a so-called Latin square. The field was divided into a given number of rows and columns. Experimental allocation was performed in such a way that a treatment appeared once in each row and once each column. For example, five treatments, A, B, C, D, E could be compared in an arrangement thus:

B	A	E	D	C
C	E	B	A	D
A	C	D	E	B
D	B	A	C	E
E	D	C	B	A

In fact, exactly this design was used in an early experiment in Bettgelert forest, each row corresponding to a different altitude of planting, the columns running (roughly) from west to east and possibly reflecting different degrees of exposure to the prevailing wind. The letters correspond to five different varieties of conifer.[9]

However, this is not the only possible arrangement subject to the restriction that a treatment shall appear once in each column and once in each row. The question then was how should one choose the particular arrangement?

The solution that Fisher published in a paper in 1926 was that one should choose the arrangement at random from amongst those satisfying the particular restrictions one wanted to apply.[10] Fisher did much more than this, however; he also showed how to analyse such experiments. In particular with his 'analysis of variance' he showed how the total variation in results in such a field could be divided into four sources: due to rows, due to columns, due to treatments and due to error. It was the comparison of the last two that permitted one to judge whether the result of an experiment was 'significant'.

Fisher's point of view as regards experiments in general was that you could (and should if practical) balance for any factors that you were going to take account of in analysis. However, once this aim had been achieved, then you should let chance decide how the treatments should be allocated to the units. An application of this philosophy to clinical trials might be as follows. Suppose that we have a placebo-controlled clinical trial of an active treatment in asthma in which forced expiratory volume in one second (FEV_1) is our outcome measure. We believe that males have higher FEV_1 values, other things being equal, than females and we would like to balance the trial by sex. We might then run two randomisation lists, one for females and one for males. (Indeed, this is what Bradford Hill did in his steptomycin trial.) In each list males and females would be allocated in equal numbers to placebo and treatment but otherwise at random. (Actually, this would require agreeing a number of each sex to be recruited onto the trial and is not always desirable, as we shall see in Chapter 5.) Fisher's philosophy would then require us to split the sources of variation into three: due to sex, due to treatment and 'random' variation. The significance of the treatment would be judged by comparing the last two sources of variation and randomisation would ensure that if there was no treatment effect, these last two sources would be expected to be comparable (once appropriately scaled).

Fisher's tea test

To illustrate another virtue of randomisation we divert to a famous experiment that Fisher described in his book of 1935, *The Design of Experiments*. 'A lady declares that by tasting a cup of tea made with milk she can discriminate whether the milk or the tea was first added to the cup.' Fisher considers an experiment in which four cups of each kind, milk in first (M) or tea in first (T) are presented to the lady in random fashion and, without knowing which is which, she has to identify them correctly. Fisher also insists that the lady shall be *told* that there will be four cups of each kind, a point that has been overlooked in some commentaries.

The experiment described is based upon a real incident.[11] The lady in question was Dr. Muriel Bristol, an algologist at Rothamsted. Fisher is supposed to have drawn a cup from the urn at teatime and offered it to her. She refused, saying that she preferred milk in first.[12] Fisher claimed that it made no difference but she insisted it did. William Roach, who was present and was later to marry Dr. Bristol, proposed testing her and a trial was arranged, although probably not exactly as described by Fisher a dozen years later.

Suppose that the lady guesses all the cups correctly. This is the most extreme result in support of her claim. We thus have a situation that is very similar to Arbuthnot's test of significance. However, the probability calculation has to proceed rather differently. The lady knows that there will be four cups of each sort. Under the null hypothesis that the lady is guessing at random, therefore, she simply needs to guess the correct sequence in which the cups are presented. How many such sequences are there?

The infernal triangle

This sort of problem is a very old one and of the kind which the mathematicians of the seventeenth century studied extensively. Blaise Pascal, whose correspondence with Nicholas Fermat in 1654 regarding problems posed by the Chevalier de Méré is often taken as the year zero for the history of probability, wrote a famous treatise on it in that year. In his honour we now refer to 'Pascal's Triangle', which is an arithmetic and geometric construction that gives the requisite answer. As dictated by *Stigler's Law of Eponomy*,[13] which states that if a discovery is named after someone he did not discover it, Pascal, is not, of course, the *discoverer* of Pascal's triangle. It was certainly known to several European mathematicians of the sixteenth century, Arab scholars knew the binomial theorem, to which it is linked, as early as the thirteenth century,[14] and the Hindu mathematicians knew the general rule by the middle of the twelfth century, whereas Pascal's Traité du triangle arithmétique was written in 1654.[15]

Nevertheless, Edwards, in his scholarly book on the subject, shows that Pascal was the first to provide a serious mathematical treatment of the properties of the triangle and to show its relevance to various important mathematical questions, including problems in probability and claims, 'That the Arithmetical Triangle should bear Pascal's name cannot be disputed'.[16] 'Pascal's' triangle is reproduced below.

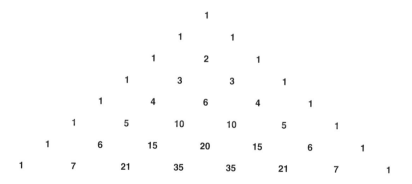

The triangle's construction is that each entry is the sum of those two elements that are the closest diagonally above it. This construction can be continued forever. The triangle's utility is that each row describes a number of trials of a 'binary' outcome, such as heads or tails, alive or dead, milk in first or tea in first. If we number the rows of the triangle starting at zero then the row number indicates the number of trials being performed. If we count in from the beginning of the row, allowing that the first element again corresponds to zero, then the number of the element gives the number of ways that you can obtain the requisite number of 'successes' in the requisite number of trials. For example, the row corresponding to 4 trials is the row

1   4   6   4   1

there is only one way that you can obtain no successes, there are four ways that you can obtain one success, there are six ways that you can obtain two successes and so forth. (These sequences were listed in Chapter 2 when discussing Arbuthnot's test.)

In general, if we have n trials and r successes, the formula that gives the requisite entry in Pascal's triangle is

$$\frac{n!}{r!(n-r)!}$$

where $n!$ (pronounced 'n factorial') is $n \times (n-1) \times (n-2) \times \cdots 2 \times 1$, so that, for example, $4! = 4 \times 3 \times 2 \times 1 = 24$ and, by special (and curious, but mathematically consistent) convention, $0! = 1$.

Now return to the Lady tasting tea. If there are four cups of each kind, then the number of sequences is the same as the number of ways that you can obtain four heads in eight tosses of a coin. That is to say that for every sequence tea in first, milk in first and so forth, there is a corresponding sequence head, tail, etc. Thus, Pascal's triangle applies and we need to substitute 8 for n and 4 for r. It turns out that $8!$ is 40 320 and dividing this twice by $4! = 24$ (one for r and once for $n - r$) we obtain 70 possible sequences.

The reason that this formula works is as follows. Suppose that we labelled each of the cups uniquely on the base using one of the letters A, B, C, D, E, F, G or H and mixed the cups up. What is the probability that the lady could guess the sequence of cups correctly? She has eight chances of getting the first cup right. Having got this right, she only has seven remaining choices for the second cup. If she gets this right there are only six choices remaining and so forth. She thus has one chance in 8 × 7 × 6 × ⋯ 2 × 1 = 8! of getting the choice right. Now suppose, however, that A, B, E and G are 'milk in first cups' and the rest are tea in first. As regards guessing the *type* of cup, it makes no difference, for example, whether she guesses A rather than B or E or G. Thus the way that the cups A, B, E and G are arranged amongst themselves is irrelevant. Similarly the way that C, D, F and H are arranged amongst themselves is irrelevant. There are 4 × 3 × 2 × 1 = 4! ways of arranging the first set of cups and 4! ways of arranging the second set. There are 4! × 4! ways of arranging them altogether whilst still making sure that the same order is always maintained as regards simply whether a cup is milk in first or tea in first. Thus we need to divide the figure of 8! by the number 4! × 4! to obtain the number of sequences that are *relevantly* different.

Since 8!/(4!4!) = 70, the lady has a 1 in 70 chance of guessing the sequence correctly. If she correctly identifies each cup, then either a rare event has occurred or what she claims is true. We thus have the basis of a significance test.

Random harvest

Here the value of randomisation is clear. It helps us in blinding the experiment. It was possibly this particular advantage that Bradford Hill had in mind when adopting the procedure for the streptomycin trial. Previously, it had been popular to use a method of alternate allocation for patients whereby (say) every odd-numbered patient was given the experimental treatment and every even-numbered patient was given control. The problem with this approach was that physicians could influence the allocation by only entering a particular patient in the trial when the next free treatment was the one desired. Choosing the sequence at random and concealing the allocation gets around this difficulty.

Randomisation also means that *on average* the groups in a clinical trial are balanced as regards any prognostic factors ('covariates') that might be influential. This latter property, however, is controversial and statisticians disagree over its utility. To explain why we return to Fisher's tea-tasting.

Suppose that we choose a sequence at random for the cups and that that sequence is M T T M T M M T. The lady guesses every cup correctly. We are impressed with this result and congratulate her. She says in reply, that of course she knew we would randomise in pairs, incidentally drawing our attention to a feature that we had not noticed, namely that, if we mark the sequence off in pairs, MT/TM/TM/MT, then for any *pair* of cups one is always milk in first (M) and the other is always T in first (T). This is a chance result. We did not plan things this way. However, of the 70 sequences, 16 have this property. (This is because if we arrange the cups in four pairs we have two choices for the order of each pair and so $2 \times 2 \times 2 \times 2 = 16$ arrangements in total.) Thus we could argue that, given the lady's false assumption about how we would randomise and given that we did by chance draw a sequence of this sort, she had a 1 in 16 chance of guessing correctly. This *conditional probability* is of course less impressive than the 1 in 70 that we previously calculated.

However, we need not have drawn a sequence randomised in pairs. In fact there are $70 - 16 = 54$ sequences that do *not* satisfy this property. We thus have a $^{54}/_{70}$ chance of drawing such a 'non-pair' sequence. Given the lady's false assumption and such a draw, then, if all is guesswork, she has zero chance of guessing the sequence correctly. Thus, before the trial starts, we have 16 chances out of 70 of drawing the sort of sequence that will lead her to have a 1 in 16 chance of guessing correctly and 54 chances out of 70 of drawing a sequence that leaves her with no chance at all. (Given her false assumption.) Putting all this together her *unconditional* probability of guessing correctly is $\left(^{16}/_{70} \times ^{1}/_{16}\right) + \left(^{54}/_{70} \times 0\right) = ^{1}/_{70}$ after all.

We now come to a controversial point in statistics. Is this *unconditional* probability relevant? It is a probability that applies before seeing the result of the randomisation and before learning that the lady had made a false assumption about the randomisation. That being so, surely it is yesterday's dregs and not currently relevant. Nearly all Bayesians and many frequentists would take the point of view that this unconditional probability is irrelevant and that we have to 'condition' on the evidence actually obtained. However, some frequentists would not agree and would regard the unconditional probability as being the relevant one.

This is where the value of Fisher's procedure reveals itself. He makes it quite explicit that the Lady must be told how the randomisation will be performed. That being so, she knows that the randomisation is not restricted to the 16 possible sequences of 4 pairs but includes all 70 sequences of 4 of each kind. Hence, there is no point in her guessing the randomisation *process*; it is known. It is only the *allocation* that is unknown. The consequence of this is that the conditional and unconditional probabilities are the same and an inferential problem is finessed.

The consolation of the marathon experimenter

The physicist and the chemist may be able to perform experiments using homogenous material and even the biologist can use genetically pure mice but the clinical scientist, like the agronomist, has to accept variability. Just as plots of land differ in fertility, patients suffering from a given disease may vary considerably in symptoms and eventual course of the disease. The only guarantee that randomisation appears to offer when constructing treatment groups is that of an irrelevant long run: 'the consolation of the marathon experimenter'. On average, over all possible randomisations, the groups will be equal.

Is this a comfort? If we are 35 000 ft above mid-Atlantic, all four engines are on fire and the captain has had a heart-attack, can we console ourselves with the thought that on average air travel is very safe? No. Nor would R. A. Fisher expect us to. We would be faced with what he referred to as 'a recognisable subset', a rather unpleasant one in this case. Fisher never intended that randomisation should exclude your taking other precautions as regards design. As already explained, he suggested, in fact, that you should balance designs for what you believed to be relevant and then randomise subject to these restrictions. Fisher also pioneered the use of models that allowed you to adjust for any imbalance after the event.

Such models will be mentioned in subsequent chapters but a simple illustration of the way they work can be given by considering the case of sex. Suppose we have randomised but *not* balanced by sex and we notice that the split is 80 males and 20 females in the active treatment group and 70 males and 30 females in the placebo group. Since, as we have already noted, other things being equal, females tend to have a lower FEV_1 than males, if we do not take account of this, the results will be biased in favour of the active treatment. We can deal with this quite simply, however, by calculating the difference between the mean of the 80 males in the treatment group and the mean of the 70 males in the placebo group, and the corresponding difference for females. Each of these two differences is an estimate of the treatment effect for the corresponding sex. It is often plausible, given a suitable choice of measurement scale, to believe that this effect does not differ too much from one group to another. (This does not require that males have similar FEV_1 values to females but simply that the *difference* that a drug makes to this measure will be similar for males and females.) It thus becomes useful to form an average of these two treatment estimates. There is a further complication whose details we cannot discuss but whose general sense can be understood. Since we have unequal numbers of males and females in the trial overall, in forming our overall average it is appropriate to give more weight to the male results. The precise value of the relative weight of male and female results is covered by an appropriate statistical theory.

However, not all relevant factors are known to us, and it is here that randomisation reveals its value. If we haven't observed a relevant factor, we can neither balance for it nor adjust for it. What Fisher showed was that randomisation meant that we could measure the variability that this uncertainty would introduce into our estimates if we randomised. If a prognostic factor varied amongst members of the trial, the results within groups would tend to be variable. It turns out that a suitable function of this variability within groups predicts how much the results between groups ought to vary. Provided we have randomised, not only are the two contributions (within and between groups) of the variable factor expected to be the same (over all randomisations) but a suitable theory, due to Fisher himself, predicts with what probability their ratio could differ by any given amount. A 'large' ratio of between-group to within-group variability then suggests that either a rare event has happened or that something else (for example a treatment effect) is causing the results from the two groups to be different. Again we have the basic argument of a significance test.

Of course, we could argue, that once again we are relying on the property of an average. However, here the property of the average *is* appropriate. Return to our example of air travel. Provided neither the person seeking insurance nor the insurer knows of any way in which a particular aircraft differs from any other, it is perfectly logical for the insurer to use the (small) probability of a crash on an 'average flight' as the basis for setting the premiums. This is true even though it is known that there is no such thing as an average flight: most end safely and a very few do not.

Ration roulette

Many clinical scientists have come to adopt randomisation as a valuable tool for clinical trials. The scientific argument is largely accepted. For those who regarded unconditional probabilities (averaged over all possible randomisations) as relevant, there was never any difficulty with randomisation. Those who consider that conditional probabilities are more relevant have more cause for scepticism, but, given that other features of design and analysis can deal with the effect of covariates, they have accepted that at the very least randomisation is harmless and may also have value in promoting 'utmost good faith'. Consider, for example, a pharmaceutical sponsor running a clinical trial. The results will have to be presented to the regulator. Included will be information, patient by patient, on relevant covariates; for example, in a trial of hypertension, we might have sex, age and baseline diastolic and systolic blood pressure. It may also have been agreed beforehand that these will be included, in addition to treatment given, in any analysis of the results. However, it would always be conceivable that the sponsor might have manipulated allocation using some further covariate measured, but not reported, in order to give the experimental treatment an advantage. Randomisation reassures the regulator that this has not happened.

However, if there is little scientific objection to randomisation amongst clinical researchers, the same is not true regarding ethics. It is felt by many to be repugnant that patients should be entered onto a clinical trial and have their treatment decided at random. A point of view that is often propounded is that a doctor entering a patient onto a randomised clinical trial should be in 'equipoise': perfectly indifferent as to which treatment is better. This view has led to a further Bayesian criticism of randomised clinical trials on grounds of ethics.

The argument goes like this. Even if we accept that from the purely scientific point of view it might be preferable to continue to randomise patients concurrently to experimental and standard treatments, having started in equipoise, it is highly likely that a point will be reached where we have a hunch that one treatment is better than another. Once we have reached this point, if we continue to randomise, we are sacrificing the interests of current patients to those of future patients. This is to treat patients as means and not ends and is unethical.[17]

Sometimes it is not possible for us to treat all patients. It has been claimed of A. B. Hill's streptomycin trial that there was not enough of the drug to treat all potentially eligible patients. A limited supply had been obtained from the United States. It thus seemed ethically acceptable to decide at random who amongst a group of otherwise eligible subjects should receive the drug.

Nevertheless, these cases are rare. It might thus seem that clinical trials as actually practised involve doctors acting against their patients' best interests. A common defence is to appeal to the so-called uncertainty principle. This maintains that randomisation is acceptable so long as the doctor is 'substantially uncertain' as to which is the best treatment. However, it is difficult to see what numerical or practical interpretation could ever be agreed for 'substantially uncertain'.

Dealing the drugs

In the context of drug development an alternative defence is possible. Since the experimental treatment being investigated is usually unlicensed, the only hope a patient may have of getting the treatment is to enter the trial. A physician who believes that the experimental treatment is better may thus say to a would-be patient: 'in this trial you will either get the standard treatment you would get anyway by entering the trial or be given a treatment that I myself expect will be superior, although I do not know that this is the case, it being the purpose of the trial to discover if this is so'.

Under these circumstances the trial may continue until one of two things happens. Either the regulator becomes convinced that the new treatment is, after all, efficacious and the treatment is granted a license, or the investigators become convinced that the treatment does not, after all, represent a therapeutic advance.

The question then arises, however, if it is only the regulator's prohibition that renders the physician's experimentation ethical then by what right does the regulator forbid? An answer to this may be found by using the device of 'the original position' employed by the philosopher John Rawls (1921–2002) in his *Theory of Justice*.[18] Rawls asks what is a just society and answers that it is one we would be happy to join if in the 'original position'. In such a position we neither know what place in the society we will have nor what gifts and disabilities.

We can use the same device in judging whether clinical trials are ethical. We must not make ethical judgements at the point of sickness only. This condemns us to take a short-term view of matters that is false. Consider a related ethical problem. How much of the general substance of society should we spend on health? If we compare the needs of an elderly person awaiting a hip replacement with those of a young fit person who wants to go on holiday, it seems clear that the former is in greater need than the latter. It is thus unethical to allow people to have holidays as long as some are waiting for hip replacements. We should arrange taxation to make sure that these ethical problems are removed. Now, however, consider the point in the original position. Which sort of a society do you want to be born into? One in which you are allowed holidays when young but you may have to wait for a hip replacement when elderly, or one in which holidays are impossible but hip replacements are guaranteed for all octogenarians?

Similarly, it is obvious that a patient awaiting a clinical trial would almost always prefer *not* to have the treatment drawn at random unless motivated by civic spirit. For suppose that A and B are being compared and that A is the standard treatment whereas B is not generally available. The patient is persuaded to enter the trial because the physician believes that B is superior, the patient trusts the physician and the trial represents the only chance of getting B. That being so, the patient would clearly prefer the certainty of getting B to the chance. Thus the regulator appears to be acting against the patient's interest.

The point is, however, that the regulator is not necessarily acting against the patient's interest in the original position. A society in which treatments are tried and rationally tested may be preferable to us all as potential patients than one in which the latest fad or hunch is tried out. After all the current generation of patients will benefit from the trials that have been performed on others.

A good red herring

But honest Doctor, wouldn't the patients have gotten better anyway? Wasn't it maybe a post-hoc, propter hoc? *Have they experimented on a whole slew of patients together, with controls?*

Sinclair Lewis, *Arrowsmith*

This still appears to leave the placebo in limbo. We can justify the use of randomised trials comparing experimental treatments to standard control ones, on the grounds that no patient receives a treatment that is believed inferior. Where the control group is given a placebo this appears not to be the case.

In fact, the use of a placebo does not in itself imply that effective treatment is being withheld. Many clinical trials are run as 'add-ons'. That is to say that where there is a (partially) effective remedy this is not withheld from patients but they are randomised to receive either the experimental treatment or its placebo as well. A placebo, being devised to match a treatment in appearance, taste, feel and so forth, is always specific to that treatment. The strategy of an add-on is very common in cancer therapy. If the new treatment proves particularly effective and there is then believed to be some potential advantage in removing the previous standard treatment, then the trial may be followed by an elimination trial. The first trial was of the form *experimental + standard* versus *'placebo to experimental' + standard*. The second will be of the form *experimental + 'placebo to standard'* versus *experimental + standard*. This second trial may take place ethically provided that the physicians running the trial believe that the new regime (with previous standard therapy eliminated) will bring advantages.

The diceman and the ethicist

Consideration of ethics seems to be getting further and further away from the role of statistics. In fact, no serious consideration of ethics can take place without taking account of what statistics has to say about designs as will now be explained with the help of an alternative to the randomised trial that has been proposed as sometimes ethically superior.

It will often be the case that patients suffering from a disease will differ considerably as regards the severity of their medical condition. For example, hypertension can be mild, moderate or severe. Under such circumstances it has been maintained that it may be unethical to consider exposing all patients to the experimental treatment. It is argued that if a partially effective treatment already exists, then this, if not ideal, will at least be adequate for all but the severely ill. Since all untried treatments carry with them a risk of side-effects, it will not be ethically acceptable to expose all patients to the risk of a side-effect as would be the case in a randomised trial. Only those who are severely ill and currently unsatisfactorily treated should be prepared to run the risk of the new treatment.

Under such circumstances, a trial that has been proposed as an ethical alternative is the so-called *regression discontinuity design* (RDD).[19] Here the mild cases serve as the control group, being given the standard treatment and the severely ill are the experimental group, given the new treatment. Obviously such a trial requires careful analysis. A randomised clinical trial is an experiment that any damn fool can analyse and frequently does, but to analyse an RDD you need a decent mathematical model. A common assumption would be that, but for the intervention, the relationship between outcome and baseline measure would be linear. Parallel lines for this relationship are then fitted for the two groups. These lines then show a difference that is postulated to exist between patients given one treatment or the other for any given values of the baseline and this is our estimate of the effect of treatment.

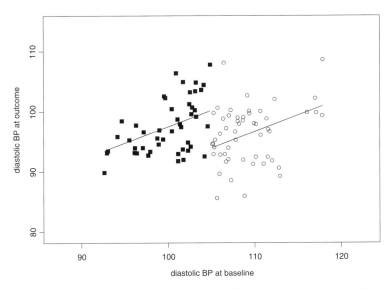

Figure 3.1 Diastolic blood pressure (mmHg) at baseline and outcome for a regression discontinuity trial. Solid squares represent patients in the control group and open circles those in the experimental group.

Figure 3.1 gives simulated data for a trial in hypertension using this approach. Patients have been sorted at baseline according to whether their diastolic blood pressure is in excess of 105 mmHg. If not they are given a standard treatment; if it is, they are given an experimental treatment. The figure plots values at outcome of the trial against values at baseline. The control group values are represented by solid squares and the experimental group values by open circles. There is little to choose between these two groups in terms of average value at outcome (vertical position). However, the point is that given the general sort of relationship between outcome and baseline illustrated by the two straight lines (which have been fitted by 'multiple regression') the values in the experimental group are lower at outcome than one would expect given how high they are at baseline. If the treatments were identical, the two lines would meet in the middle. The extent to which they do not is an estimate of the treatment effect.

Obviously the validity of the conclusion is heavily dependent on the presumed model. There is a further disadvantage, however. Statistical theory shows that, even if the model is correct, at least 2.75 times as many patients are required to produce an answer which has the same precision as that of a randomised clinical trial.[20] This lower bound is reached when it is the case that the severely ill form half of all patients. In what follows, this will be assumed to be the case.

Now suppose that we accept the argument that only the severely ill patients should run the risk of trying the experimental treatment. This ethical requirement does not prevent our allocating the standard treatment to them. In fact, if we don't run the trial this is what they will get as, indeed will all patients in regions other than that in which the trial is being run. We could thus run an RCT in which we only recruited severely ill patients, allocating half the standard treatment and half the experimental one. Suppose that we decide to make absolutely no use of the results from the moderately ill patients in doing this, and suppose, for argument's sake, that we randomise 100 patients to each of the two treatment groups making 200 in total. If the alternative to this approach is the RDD, we shall have to have at least 275 severely ill patients given experimental treatment with 275 moderately ill given the control. This means that, other things being equal, we shall finish the randomised trial earlier. If the experimental treatment is not proved superior we shall have allocated 175 more severely ill patients inappropriately to experimental treatment using the RDD. If the experimental treatment is proved superior after all, we shall of course have treated 100 severely ill patients with the standard treatment using the RCT and this may be considered a potential loss. On the other hand, if the experimental treatment is eventually to be used for the moderately ill, and it is hard to see how they can be considered an adequate control group if this possibility is excluded, then 275 moderately ill patients will have been given an inferior treatment with the RDD. Although, during the time the RCT has been running only 200 moderately ill patients have been suffering this loss, a difference of 75 to the benefit of the RCT compared to the RDD. Thus, the net loss under these circumstances in running an RCT compared to an RDD is $100 - 75 = 25$. Hence, the RCT treats 25 patients sub-optimally compared to the RDD if the experimental treatment is eventually proved superior. Then again, if the control treatment is eventually proved superior the RDD treats 175 patients sub-optimally compared to the RCT. This disadvantage in terms of potential losses of 175:25 or 7:1 makes it hard to claim the RDD as being ethically superior.

Two morals can be drawn from this example. First, the relevance of statistical considerations to the ethics of clinical trials. Second, that although the RCT may seem morally repugnant, it is more difficult to produce ethically superior alternatives than may be supposed at first sight.

Dynamic allocation

This does not mean that statistics exonerates the RCT compared to all possible alternatives. In fact, if we do not make an artificial distinction between patients in the trial and those who will be treated in the future, then a radically different approach to clinical trials suggests itself.

Suppose that we have a very rare disease and are aware that medical progress makes it highly unlikely that any new treatment that we discover to be superior to a standard will remain the 'best' for very long. It is then quite possible that the patients that we treat in a clinical trial will form a large proportion of those who could ever be treated with the new treatment. A randomised clinical trial does not then seem a very attractive option. To take the argument to extremes, suppose that we are faced with a single patient only and believe that no others will follow. There is no point in deciding this patient's treatment at random; we might as well back our best hunch.

One way of proceeding might be as follows. We regard the treatment of each patient as being determined by two, possibly conflicting, forces. One is to do the best we can for him or her on the basis of existing knowledge. The other is to treat the patient in such a way that the information gained will be of greatest use in treating future patients. These two will not always agree. Suppose that we are comparing two treatments A and B and currently assess their 'cure rates' as being 0.3 and 0.4 respectively. Our belief suggests that it is in the interest of the next patient to treat him or her with B. But now suppose that B's cure probability is fairly precisely estimated, being based on treatment with a large number of cases, but that of A is not well estimated. The possibility then remains open that the true cure rate with A is much higher than the value of 0.3 we currently assign to it. It would be in the interest of future patients to have this doubt resolved just in case, contrary to current impressions, the true cure rate of A is, in fact, higher than that of B. Thus, it would be best for this purpose to assign the next patient to treatment A.

Using a Bayesian approach and applying functions that trade-off the value of future against current cures, it is possible to develop algorithms which assign patients dynamically in a way that is 'optimal'. These designs have been extensively investigated by the Bayesian statistician Don Berry and his co-workers.[21] The conclusions of their research is that the RCT is not too bad in terms of this philosophy provided that the disease is not rare and provided that the discount function used for comparing short-term against long-term gains is not too severe.

The RCT today

Despite being the subject of frequent criticism as being inhuman or irrational, the RCT is thriving, at least if numbers are any judge. For example, at the time of writing this chapter (May 2002) the Centerwatch Clinical Trials Listing Service, list 41 000 pharmaceutical industry and research council sponsored clinical trials in the United States alone. It is generally estimated that the number of randomised clinical trials that have now been run must be measured in the hundreds of thousands. For example, The Cochrane Collaboration, an organisation devoted to synthesising evidence from clinical trials and whose work we shall encounter in Chapter 8, lists more than 300 000 on its database. Indeed, in the context of drug regulation, it is almost impossible to get any treatment accepted unless it has been tested in randomised clinical trials. Drug regulation in the United States, the European Union and Japan is conducted according to a set of principles agreed by the International Conference on Harmonisation. These principles are also used by many other countries. Guideline E10 (E stands for efficacy) on Choice of Control Group and Related Issues in Clinical Trials, although it does not rule out external controls, makes it clear that in general only randomised clinical trials will be regarded as providing acceptable evidence of efficacy.[22]

We shall return to clinical trials to look seriously at a potential problem of interpretation in Chapter 5. For the moment, however, it is time that we turned to considering some more fundamental difficulties facing the medical statistician – some problems of statistical inference itself.

4

Of dice and men*

Tossing and turning*

Which is more likely in tossing a fair coin ten times, that you alternately get head, tail, head, tail and so forth, or that you get ten heads in a row? Let us calculate. For the alternating series we have half a chance of getting a head and then half a chance of getting a tail and then half a chance of getting a head and so forth. So the overall probability of this series is $(1/2)^{10} = 1/2^{10} = 1/1024$. On the other hand, the chance of getting ten heads in a row is one-half times a half times a half, and so forth, and equals $(1/2)^{10} = 1/2^{10} = 1/1024$. In other words, the two events are equally likely, or, as it turns out, unlikely.

Did you think that the sequence corresponding to head tail head and so forth would be more likely? Perhaps you were thinking of a related problem? *Which is more likely in tossing a fair coin ten times, that you get five heads and five tails in any order or that you get ten heads in a row?* Here the point is that there are many more sequences that satisfy the condition of five heads and five tails than the alternating one originally defined. Pascal's triangle tells us how many, or alternatively the corresponding formula, which gives $10!/(5!5!) = 252$. So the probabilities are now $252/1024$ and $1/1024$. The probability of getting five heads and five tails in any order is 252 times as great as that of getting ten heads in a row.

So far so elementary, so far so obvious, you may say, nothing very surprising in this. However, for what appears to be a very similar situation, this ratio of probabilities is 252 times too large. We can easily define a problem for which the probability of getting five heads and five tails *in any order* in ten tosses of a coin is the same as the probability of getting ten heads in a row, despite the fact that there are 252 ways of obtaining the former result and only one way of obtaining the latter.

Consider a very slight change to the original question. *Which is more likely in tossing a coin ten times, that you alternately get head, tail, head, tail and so forth, or that you get ten heads in a row?* This question is identical to the first one except that the word *fair* has been removed. A frequentist faced with this question will reply that it cannot be answered. There is a piece of knowledge that is missing, namely the probability that the coin will come up 'heads' in a single toss of a coin. The Bayesian also cannot answer this question as put, because it implies that the probability is a property of the coin and the event alone. As we have seen, for Bayesians probability is a matter of belief. It is personal, a property of the subject as well as the object. However what we *can* ask is the sort of question a Bayesian fundamentalist, a Calvinist of probability, a holder of the unswerving, the pure, the true faith that salvation comes through belief alone, can always answer. *What odds would* you *offer, in tossing a coin, on getting ten heads in a row rather than head tail head tail and so forth?*

In the extreme subjective form of Bayesianism that is now fashionable, this sort of question is always answerable. Given an assumption of independence, it simply requires a prior belief in every possible degree of bias in the coin being tossed. Suppose that we take the case that Laplace considers: that of complete ignorance; we can then apply Laplace's rule of succession. It turns out that that the following theorem applies.

If *your* probability that the next time *you* toss a coin it comes up heads obeys Laplace's law of succession, then *your* probability of obtaining *any* given number of heads in n tosses of the coin is $1/(n + 1)$.

We are now going to prove this using an approach known as *mathematical induction*. That is to say we are going to do the following:

1.   Prove that *if* it is true for n tosses of a coin it is true for $n + 1$ tosses.
2.   Prove that it *is* true for one toss.

Now if point 1 is true then given point 2 it also holds for two tosses of a coin from which it follows that it holds for three tosses and hence for four tosses and so forth. Is the principle of this clear? Let us proceed to the proof.

Suppose that the theorem is true and we have tossed a coin n times and observed X heads, where X (obviously) is a number less than or equal to n. The theorem says that the probability of obtaining X heads is $1/(n + 1)$. For example, if X is any number between 0 and 7 and n is 7, the probability of X is $1/8$. Now consider first a special case: that of obtaining $n + 1$ heads in $n + 1$ tosses. To obtain this we must have had n heads in the first n tosses. Laplace's law of succession says that the probability that the *next* toss comes up heads is $(n + 1)/(n + 2)$. However, we have just said that we are going to assume that our theorem holds, from which it follows that the probability of the first n tosses being heads is $1/(n + 1)$. If we multiply this by $(n + 1)/(n + 2)$, we obtain the probability that the first n tosses are heads and so is toss $n + 1$. The answer is $1/(n + 2)$. But this is just the answer from our theorem with $n + 1$ substituted for n. Hence, in this special case, if the theorem holds for n it holds for $n + 1$. The case of no heads ($n + 1$ tails) can be dealt with identically by replacing the word 'heads' with 'tails' in the above and vice versa.

Now let us consider the more general case of how we can get X heads in $n + 1$ tosses of a coin where X is greater than zero and less than $n + 1$. Well clearly we either have $X - 1$ heads in the first n tosses and then obtain a head on toss $n + 1$ or we have X heads in the first n tosses and then obtain a tail. Consider the second situation. *Given* that we have X heads in n tosses, we clearly have $(n - X)$ tails. Laplace's law of succession says that the probability of the next toss being a tail is $[(n - X) + 1]/(n + 2)$. The probability of the first n tosses showing X heads and the next toss showing a tail is thus the product of this probability and the value of $1/(n + 1)$ that we are assuming from the theorem. This product is thus $[(n - X) + 1]/[(n + 1)(n + 2)]$. On the other hand, if we have $X - 1$ heads so far, then Laplace's law of succession says that the probability of the next toss being a head is $[(X - 1) + 1]/(n + 2)$ and when we multiply this by the assumed probability of $1/(n + 1)$ we get $X/[(n + 1)(n + 2)]$. Adding the two probabilities together and noticing that the X terms cancel we obtain $(n + 1)/[(n + 1)(n + 2)] = 1/(n + 2)$. Note that this answer does not depend on X. In other words it is the same however many heads are specified to be obtained.

We have now secured the first part of our proof, namely that if the theorem holds for n tosses it holds for $n + 1$ tosses, for, starting with the probability of $1/(n + 1)$ for n tosses, we obtain $1/(n + 2)$ for $n + 1$ tosses which is the same formula with $n + 1$ substituted for n. The second part of the proof is trivial. We prove it is true for $n = 1$. But Laplace's law of succession simply yields $1/2$ for the probability of 'heads' on the first toss of a coin and also

$1/_2$ for 'tails'. These are the only two possible sequences, each is equally likely and, since $n = 1$, then according to our theorem, the probability of each is equal to $1/(n + 1) = 1/_2$. Hence our theorem is proved.

Now return to the problem with ten tosses. The theorem says that *your* probability of obtaining ten heads in a row is $1/_{11}$ and that *your* probability of five heads in any order is also $1/_{11}$. But, there are 252 ways that we can obtain five heads in any order, only one of which is the alternating sequence head, tail, head, tail, etc. so that *your* probability of obtaining this sequence is not the same as *your* probability of obtaining the sequence of ten heads, the ratio of the latter to the former probability being 252.

The bliss of ignorance

This may seem rather surprising. If we *know* the coin is fair, the probabilities of the two sequences arising are equal. If we know nothing about the coin, Laplace says our probabilities vary by a ratio of 252 to 1. It is important to appreciate, however, that this result relies on assuming that every possible probability for the coin is equally likely. This was mentioned in Chapter 2, although we did not prove it. However, we are now in a better position to understand it.

Imagine that we toss the coin 999 998 times and we intend to apply Laplace's law of succession to the probability of obtaining a head. Now consider the probabilities that we will issue for the result of tossing the coin the 999 999th time. Remember that to apply Laplace's law we imagine we already have observed one head and one tail before we start, to which we add the observed results using the ratio as our probability. Thus the lowest possible probability we will issue will be 1/1 000 000 (if we have had no heads) and the highest will be 999 999/1 000 000 (if we have had 999 998 heads). The other possible values are the 999 997 values that lie at intervals of 1/1 000 000 between these two. Laplace's rule also implies that each of these 999 999 values has equal probability.

Now suppose that we are required to bet at the beginning as to whether our probability statement for the 999 999th toss once we have completed 999 998 will be less than or equal to some given value q, where q lies between 0 and 1. Laplace's rule tells us that this probability must be very close to q. In fact it can differ from q by no more than 1/1 000 000, this difference depending upon how close to one of the *exact* possible probability values q is.

If we are worried about this possible discrepancy of 1/1 000 000 we can let the number of tosses grow to a billion, a thousand billion and so forth. If we use Laplace's rule, our *forecast* at the beginning of the series as to whether we will issue a probability statement at the end that is less than or equal to q will be extremely close to q, whatever the value of q is. However, we are Bayesians. We do not need Laplace's rule to issue probability forecasts; we can use introspection instead. The result of this introspection will be to assign a value of q to the probability that we will forecast q or less for all possible q at the end of our 1000 billion tosses, only if we regard every value of q as equally likely. Hence Laplace's rule corresponds to this equiprobable position, the position of prior ignorance.

With all this coin-tossing, the reader's head will be spinning. It is time for another historical diversion. We pause to look at David Hume and his challenge to philosophy, science and statistics in order to consider whether Laplace answered it.

The man who woke up Immanuel Kant

He said what Kant did, trying to answer Hume (to whom I say there is no answer), was to invent more and more sophisticated stuff, till he could no longer see through it and could believe it to be an answer.

J. E. Littlewood[1]

Whereas James Bernoulli and Thomas Bayes were unfortunate enough to die before their masterpieces were published, the Scottish philosopher David Hume (1711–1776) managed the unhappy trick of seeing his masterpiece die as it was born. 'Never literary attempt was more unfortunate than my Treatise of human Nature. It fell dead-born from the press . . .'.[2] However, the thump of his baby as it landed in its coffin was heard some years later in Königsberg, where it woke Immanuel Kant from his dogmatic slumbers. No doubt, many a student since has wished that Hume had let sleeping fogs lie.

Hume's masterpiece was published in 1739–1740. Considering that Hume confessed that love of literary fame was his main motivation in writing, its reception must have been particularly galling. Worse was to follow. Hume applied for the Chair of Ethics and Pneumatical Philosophy in Edinburgh. The blow of this failed application appears to have taken the wind out of his sails and he abandoned writing for a while, becoming in turn a tutor to a mad nobleman, the Marquess of Annandale and secretary to General St Claire.[3]

Hume eventually re-worked his masterpiece, in a slimmer form as *An Enquiry Concerning Human Understanding*, 1748, that he was later to regard as being the superior expression of his thought. Modern philosophers have not always agreed. However, it was in this latter form that Kant came to read him. Hume is now regarded as one of the greatest philosophers of the eighteenth century so that he has achieved a posthumous, or even post-Humes, fame of the sort he desired.

The other form of induction

Mathematical induction, which we used to prove our theorem, is a form of reasoning which makes many uneasy but which is generally accepted by mathematicians as being sound. The reason we are uneasy is that it involves a form of arguing from the particular to the general. The reason it is sound is that we provide a rule that we can see will enable us to produce *any* particular case amongst the infinity that we call general.

Consider another example. The formula for the sum of the first n integers is $n(n + 1)/2$. Assume it is true. Add the next integer, $n + 1$. The combined sum is now $n(n + 1)/2 + (n + 1) = \{n(n + 1) + 2(n + 1)\}/2 = (n^2 + 3n + 2)/2 = (n + 2)(n + 1)/2$, which is the same formula as before but with $n + 1$ substituted for n. Hence if the formula is true for the first n integers it is true for the first $n + 1$, in which case it would hold for the first $n + 2$ and so *ad infinitum*. But substituting $n = 1$ we obtain $1(1 + 1)/2 = 1$, so the formula is true for this case and hence for all the others. What we have done is to show that we can always construct a higher step in a ladder of logic and that we can also take the first one; hence, we can climb to any desired height.

Of course, the reader will no doubt remember that there is a much simpler proof of this formula. Take the first n numbers and write them in ascending order. Now write them in descending order in a line below and add them together thus:

Ascending	1	2	3	4	5	6	7	...	n
Descending	n	$n-1$	$n-2$	$n-3$	$n-4$	$n-5$	$n-6$	...	1
Total		$n+1$	$n+1$	$n+1$	$n+1$	$n+1$	$n+1$	$n+1$		$n+1$

There are n such sums equal to $n + 1$, so that the total of these sums is $n(n + 1)$. But since we have written down the numbers twice, the answer we seek is half of this and is $n(n + 1)/2$, which is the formula we had previously.

However, reassuring as this may be, it is not the point. If our proof by induction were the only proof we had, it would suffice.

Suppose, however, that instead I had offered you the following 'proof'. Applying the formula when $n = 1$, I obtain 1, which is the right answer. Applying it to $n = 2$, I obtain 3, which, since $1 + 2 = 3$, is the right answer. Again, applying it to $n = 3$, I obtain 6, which, since $1 + 2 + 3 = 6$, is the right answer and so forth. I carry on for a long while in this vein obtaining answers that always confirm the formula. Eventually we all get exhausted and agree that the formula is correct.

This is clearly not good enough by the standards of mathematical proof. On the other hand, to the extent that we regard scientific laws as having been proved, they seem to have been proved in this sort of way. We propose a law and find that when applied under all sorts of circumstances it predicts the phenomena we observe and it doesn't make any false predictions so we assume that it is true. This is called scientific induction.

It is Hume's realisation that induction is problematic that is responsible for his own induction into the philosopher's pantheon. As Hume puts it, 'The idea of cause and effect is deriv'd from experience, which presenting us with certain objects constantly conjoin'd with each other, produces such a habit of surveying them in that relation, that we cannot without a sensible violence survey them in any other.'[4] But, as Hume shows, this habit of association is not logical. Hume's paradox of induction can be expressed like this.

1. Scientific knowledge is acquired by rational means only.
2. Induction is necessary for acquiring scientific knowledge.
3. Induction is not rational.

Each of these statements appears plausible taken alone. However, they are an incompatible set. This is the paradox of scientific induction.

Baron reasoning

Does Baron Laplace have the answer? Perhaps his law of succession can come to the rescue. In fact, Laplace famously, and perhaps not entirely seriously, calculated the probability that the Sun would rise tomorrow based on it having risen so far for a number of years.[5]

Return to our formula for the sum of the first n numbers. Clearly the formula applies in some cases and we have found none in which it does not apply. Suppose we have tried it out for 100 different values of n and suppose that we consider that before having tried any values whatsoever, the probability that the law would hold in any one case could be described by the principle of insufficient reason. Laplace's law of succession says that the probability that it applies to the next case we shall encounter is 101/102. This seems fairly large, and although it is less than satisfactory in the particular context of mathematics, perhaps in the context of empirical science it will do. We can never be absolutely certain but we can be pretty certain given a large case of positive instances of the law applying and no counter-examples.

There are two serious problems with this point of view. To explain what the first is, we divert to consider a famous Bayesian.

Sir Harold Jeffreys (1891–1989)

Harold Jeffreys was born in Fatfield County Durham, a village that is associated with the medieval legend of the Lambton Worm.[6] Having already obtained an ordinary degree from a college of Durham University he went to Cambridge in 1910 to read mathematics where he attended St. Johns. He graduated a Wrangler in 1913, the year after R. A. Fisher.[7] Apart from a brief rainy spell at the Meteorological Office, 1917–1922, he spent all of his very long and sunny career at Cambridge. His interests covered geophysics, astronomy and hydrodynamics but also probability theory and scientific inference, and were thus very similar, making due allowances for a difference of nearly two centuries, to those of Daniel Bernoulli.

Jeffreys's considerable reputation depends not only on his contribution to statistics but also on his work as a geophysicist, although in this context, he is often unfortunately remembered for his opposition to the theory of continental drift. (R. A. Fisher, who knew Jeffreys well and was on cordial terms with him despite differing in his views on statistical inference, was an early believer in continental drift.[8]) Jeffreys's importance to statistics rests on his book, *Theory of Probability*, first published in 1939.

In statistical matters, Jeffreys was a Bayesian, and at a time when this was very unpopular due to the spectacular advances that R. A. Fisher and subsequently Jerzy Neyman and Egon Pearson had made in the 1920s and 1930s in developing the frequentist theory. Jeffreys's statistical reputation has grown rapidly since the 1960s as Bayesian methods have become more popular and this despite the fact that his own particular approach, although technically very interesting and on occasion useful, is increasingly regarded as philosophically unsound, even by Bayesians.

Jeffreys tried to develop the Laplacian form of Bayesianism. That is to say that although he regarded probability as a degree of belief and considered that such belief should be updated in the light of evidence using Bayes theorem, he nevertheless felt that scientists ought to agree on their beliefs. Thus his subjective probabilities were close to being objective.

The Jeffreys objection*

Nothing comes of nothing

Shakespeare, King Lear

In an article entitled, In praise of Bayes, that appeared in *The Economist* in September 2000, the unnamed author tried to show how a newborn baby could, through successively observed sunrises and the application of Laplace's law of succession, acquire increasing certainty that the Sun would always rise. As *The Economist* put it, 'Gradually, the initial belief that the Sun is just as likely as not to rise each morning is modified to become a near-certainty that the Sun will always rise'.[9] This is false: not so much praise as hype. *The Economist* had confused the probability that the Sun will rise tomorrow with the probability that it will always rise. One can only hope this astronomical confusion at that journal does not also attach to beliefs about share prices.

The importance of this distinction and a difficulty with Laplace's law of succession that it raises were pointed to by Jeffreys and is why we are interested in him here. Return to the value of 101/102 that we obtained for the probability, having had 100 successful instances and no failures, that the next time we tried to apply the law for the sum of the first n integers it will work. This, however, is the probability that it works once (that is to say next time), not the probability that it will always work. How can we calculate the probability that it will *always* work?

If Laplace's law of succession applies the answer is, 'very simply'. Take the problem of coin tossing and consider, for example, the probability before undertaking the first toss, that the first n tosses of a coin will come up heads and then the next m will come up heads. This is simply the probability that the first $n + m$ tosses will show $n + m$ heads and, using our theorem from earlier in the chapter, must be $1/(n + m + 1)$. However, this event is of course a joint event, the two constituent events being, 'the first n tosses are heads,' and 'the next m tosses are heads'. Call the first of these events, A and the second, B. We have thus established that $P(A \& B) = 1/(n + m + 1)$.

But $P(A)$ is the probability that the first n tosses are heads and, using our theorem again, equals $1/(n + 1)$. Now we can use Bayes theorem[10] to calculate the probability of B given A as $P(B \mid A) = P(B \text{ \& } A)/P(A) = [1/(n + m + 1)]/[1/(n + 1)] = (n + 1)/(n + m + 1)$.

What we have calculated is the probability that the next m tosses will be heads given that the first n were. Note that if $m = 1$, the probability is $(n + 1)/(n + 2)$, which is, of course, Laplace's law of succession, as it should be. The problem, however, which Jeffreys noted is this. Suppose that we have observed a large number of heads and no tails. This formula now applies and n is large. Although the probability that the next toss will be a head is close to one, to find the probability that *all* future tosses will show a head we have to let m grow to infinity and this makes $(n + 1)/(n + m + 1)$ approach zero. In other words the probability of *this* event is effectively zero. This may seem not unreasonable when tossing a coin but when applied to a scientific law it means that however many times we have seen it verified, the probability of its being true is zero.

It thus seems that Laplace does not answer Hume. Jeffreys has a 'solution' to the problem. This is that we have to abandon the uninformative prior that led to the law of succession. This is the origin of the problem. If this applies, each probability a priori of the coin showing heads is equally likely. This means that the probability that this probability is greater than $9/_{10}$ is $1/_{10}$. The probability that it is greater than 999 in a thousand is 1 in a thousand, than 999 999 in a million is 1 in a million and so on. Obviously this implies that the probability that the probability is exactly 1 is (effectively) zero. In the context of science, to use this form of prior implies that every scientific law has probability zero a priori. No amount of evidence can overcome this degree of scepticism. Jeffreys's solution (in the context of coin tossing) is that we have to take some of the probability we would otherwise have smeared evenly over the interval 0 to 1 and place lumps of it at each end (and possibly in the middle).

As Jeffreys puts it, 'Any clearly stated law has a positive prior probability, and therefore an appreciative posterior probability until there is definite evidence against it'.[11] With the dual devices of assigning positive prior probability to simple prior statements such as 'this coin is fair', 'this coin always shows heads', 'this coin always shows tails' and uninformative priors for remaining cases, Jeffreys hoped to rescue Laplace's programme from its difficulties. However, Bayesians with a greater enthusiasm for a more radically subjective view of probability were pointing to a problem, the second of the two difficulties to which we earlier alluded.

The subjectivists

A foolish consistency is the hobgoblin of little minds

Emerson

Jeffreys's programme was to develop a calculus of probability which, whilst recognising that probability was a measure of belief, showed how increasing evidence would force a consensus of belief that was effectively objective. However, others were working on a more radical form of Bayesianism that denied even this *necessary* degree of convergence. Some very brief sketches are included here of some of the main figures.

Frank Ramsey (1903–1930) whose father became President of Magdalene College and whose younger brother was to become Archbishop of Canterbury was educated at Winchester and Cambridge.[12] Although he died aged only 26 (of jaundice) he had already been making important contributions to mathematics, philosophy and economics when an undergraduate and had helped to translate Wittgenstein into English. In his essay Truth and Probability (1923), Ramsey demonstrates a relationship between utility and probability. A key concept he develops is that which he calls *consistency* and which modern Bayesians, following de Finetti, call *coherence*. What Ramsey shows is that although there may be no particular reason why two persons should agree in assessing the probability of events, nevertheless their assessments of sets of events must obey certain axioms. As he put it, 'If anyone's mental condition violated these laws ... He could have a book made against him by a cunning better and would then stand to lose in any event'.[13]

This particular argument is sometimes referred to as the 'Dutch book argument'. The American mathematician and statistician Jimmy Savage (1917–1971) later developed similar approaches. Savage was at Chicago, a university with an extremely powerful school of economics and which has been very influential in promoting exchanges of ideas between economists and statisticians. Savage himself collaborated on various papers with Milton Friedman, who was a statistician at one time, and his subsequent statistical thinking was strongly influenced by economic theories of utility. What Savage succeeded in doing was to relate probability to utility and vice versa by grounding them both in a theory of rational decision-making based upon the idea of coherence.[14] In Savage's approach an individual will (or ought to) act so as to maximise his or her expected utility. This requires personal probability and utility assessments. These may differ from individual to individual but must be coherent. Although he started out in the frequentist tradition, Savage was later to develop the extreme form of Bayesianism that only subjective probabilities existed, which he shared with de Finetti.

An important collaborator of Savage's was the British mathematician and statistician Dennis Lindley. Lindley was born in south London in 1923 and read mathematics at Cambridge where he eventually headed the statistical laboratory before taking up a chair at Aberystwyth. He subsequently held the Chair of Statistics at University College London in Karl Pearson's old department before taking early retirement in 1977.[15] Lindley started out in the frequentist tradition but, in an influential and productive statistical life, has had two dramatic conversions. First, to a general adoption of the Bayesian paradigm. Second, to a renunciation of the semi-objective approach of Jeffreys when logical difficulties with this were revealed in an important paper by Dawid, Stone and Zidek.[16] Lindley had been a relentless critic of frequentist procedures, pointing out bizarre features of this school of inference.

A more moderate position was held by I. Jack Good (1916–), born Isidore Jakob Gudak, son of an immigrant London shopkeeper.[17] Good was at Jesus College Cambridge before the War, completed a Ph.D. under the famous mathematician G. H. Hardy and later worked for Alan Turing in the code-breaking unit at Bletchley Park. Good was one of the pioneers in the field of computing but has also claimed that he was the only Bayesian attending Royal Statistical Society meetings during the 1950s. Good accepts that objective probabilities may exist but holds that they can only be measured with the aid of subjective probabilities.

Fascism and probability

The most extreme subjectivist view of statistical inference, however, was proposed by the Italian actuary and mathematician Bruno de Finetti (1906–1985). According to de Finetti, a serious cause of error in our thinking is the 'inveterate tendency of savages to objectivize and mythologize everything'.[18] (Not to be confused with the inveterate tendency of Savage's to subjectivise and psychologise everything.)

de Finetti was born in Innsbruck of Italian parents. He studied mathematics in Milan, graduating in 1927. After work at the National Institute of Statistics in Rome he moved to Trieste where he worked for an insurance company from 1931 to 1946, subsequently moving back to Rome where he held Chairs in economics and then probability at the University.

In a bizarre paper of 1931 entitled 'Probabilismo', he expresses not only his hatred of 'objective' probability but also of realists in general and the thrill he felt in October 1922 at the Fascist triumph. As he puts it in ending his paper, 'Those delicious absolute truths that stuffed the demo-liberal brains! That impeccable rational mechanics of the perfect civilian regime of the peoples, conforming to the rights of man and various other immortal principles! It seemed to me I could see them, these Immortal Principles, as filthy corpses in the dust. And with what conscious and ferocious voluptuousness I felt myself trampling them, marching to hymns of triumph, obscure but faithful Blackshirt'.[19]

Although he spoke German and French in addition to Italian, de Finetti's knowledge of English was poor. He was really 'discovered' for the Anglo-Saxon world by Savage (who would have been horrified by his politics), who made de Finetti's important paper on probability[20] (in French) of 1937 known to a wider audience. A student of Dennis Lindley's, Adrian Smith, collaborated to translate de Finetti's book, *Theory of Probability* (1970), into English.

de Finetti and the divergence from convergence

de Finetti's objection to any theory of *necessary* convergence of Bayesians in the light of evidence can be simply illustrated with help of a brilliant concrete illustration of his which we will modify slightly.[21] Suppose that we consider inspecting a batch of 1000 specimens for quality. We examine 100 items at random and find that 15 of them do not work but the specification says that for a batch of 1000 to be acceptable no more than 50 should be defective. What may we expect about the number of defectives in the remaining 900? In particular, for example, what can we say about the probability that the remaining 900 will contain 36 or more defectives, a number that renders the batch unacceptable?

If we attempt to apply Laplacian reasoning to this problem we might imagine that we start with some prior probability regarding the number of defectives in the batch which we can express in terms of two values a and b. The ratio of a to $(a + b)$ governs our prior belief in the proportion that is defective and the total of $(a + b)$ the extent to which our belief is modified by the evidence. For example, Jones might have $a = 0.1, b = 1.9, a + b = 2$, Smith might have $a = 1, b = 19, a + b = 20$, and Green might have $a = 0.5$, $b = 19.5, a + b = 20$. Their probability assessments that the first item drawn will be defective are $^{0.1}/_2 = 0.05$, $^1/_{20} = 0.05$, and $^{0.5}/_{20} = 0.025$.

Applying a Laplacian-type algorithm we add the number defective, 15, to the numerator and the number examined, 100, to the denominator of our probability forecasts. Thus as regards the next item examined, Smith issues $15.1/102 = 0.148$, Jones has $16/120 = 0.134$ and Green has $15.5/120 = 0.129$.

What we can see from this example is that the three Bayesians have moved close to the observed proportion of 0.15. Admittedly, Smith and Jones originally agreed perfectly as regards the probability for the next item examined and now only agree approximately but this is simply because the facts disagree with their prior opinions and Jones, having held these more strongly than Smith, has not moved as far away from them. On the other hand, Green, who disagreed originally with Smith and Jones, has now moved much closer to them. As the observations increase they will move closer together.

However, as de Finetti points out there is absolutely no obligation to use rules of this form. Consider three different cases. Case 1: we believe that batches are packed from very large production runs that have been mixed together. Case 2: batches are packed from given runs of particular machines and these tend to drift badly from their settings from time to time. Case 3: we think that the product is inspected prior to packing to ensure that no more than 50 per batch are defective. This might be the case where production costs are high, the average proportion defective is close to that which customers will tolerate and the manufacturer has a ruthless attitude to its customers.

Suppose that for all three cases we have very strong evidence that the *average* proportion defective is 4 per 100. In case 1, the fact that the first 100 had 15 defectives will be regarded as being no more informative about this batch than about production in general, about which we already have a firm opinion. Hence it is irrelevant for the remaining 900 and our probability assessment is unaffected. In case 2, we think that the high rate of defectives encountered to date is an indication that this is a bad batch. Hence the probability of any one of the remaining 900 being defective is increased. In case 3, we think that the fact that there are 15 defectives in the 100 *reduces* the probability of any given item of the remaining 900 being defective compared with the prior assessment.

What de Finetti's example shows is that convergence of opinion is not necessary for the simple reason that divergence can be perfectly logical. In other words, de Finetti accepts Hume's criticism wholeheartedly. There is no guarantee that we will iterate towards to truth. We simply have to issue bets in a way that is coherent. For example if, in tossing a coin, you believe that the probability that the next toss will show a head is $1/2$ and that the next two tosses will show a head is $1/3$, then having obtained a head on the next toss your probability that the second toss will be a head is $2/3$. This follows simply from the rule required for coherent betting. The joint probability is the product of the marginal probability and the conditional so that $1/3 = 1/2 \times 2/3$. It may be that the world is so constructed that such coherent betting also resonates with the way that laws of nature unfold. This would, indeed, be regarded as a reasonable belief by de Finetti but nothing *requires* it.

We now leave the Bayesians, to consider two non-Bayesians: first the statistician Jerzy Neyman and then the philosopher Karl Popper.

The man who was not interested in inferences

Jerzy Neyman (1894–1981) was born of Polish parents in Bendery, then part of the Russian Empire and now in Moldova. In 1912 he entered the University of Kharkov to study Physics and Mathematics. During a period of post-war hostility between the newly established Poland and Russia, Neyman was interned. It seems that one of his professors had a beautiful ballet dancer for a daughter who got involved with a Polish spy[22] and Neyman was damned by association. In 1921 an exchange of prisoners took place and Neyman went to Poland for the first time.[23] In 1923 he obtained a Ph.D. from the University of Warsaw on probabilistic problems in agriculture: the field (it seems the most appropriate word in the context) that was also claiming the attention of R. A. Fisher.

Neyman obtained a postdoctoral fellowship to study with Karl Pearson in University College London in 1924. From 1925 onwards, Neyman began an important collaboration with Egon Pearson (1895–1980), son of Karl. Their work together began in a period in which Karl Pearson's domination of the biometrics world was being increasingly challenged by the rapid advances in statistics that R. A. Fisher had been making at Rothamsted. Fisher had vastly extended the application of tests of significance and had also, as was discussed in Chapter 2, proposed the concept of likelihood. Neyman and Pearson were to discover an important connection between the two that will be discussed below in due course.

In 1934 Karl Pearson retired and his inheritance at UCL was divided between Egon and R. A. Fisher, the former taking over biometrics and the latter genetics. Neyman, who had been in Poland between 1928 and 1934, returned to UCL to join Egon. There was soon to be a falling out with Fisher. In 1935 Neyman read a paper on 'Statistical Problems in Agricultural Experimentation' to the Royal Statistical Society which corrected certain supposed errors of Fisher in dealing with the analysis of Latin squares. It was not obvious at the time but in fact Neyman was using a different (and less realistic) model to Fisher. The relationship of these two giants of twentieth century statistics never recovered from this disagreement.

In 1938, Neyman moved to Berkley in California where he was to spend the rest of his life. Mathematical statistics as practised in the USA in its frequentist form can be largely regarded as being the school of Neyman.

Of lemmas and dilemmas*

Which of your Philosophical Systems is any more than a dream-theorem; a net quotient, confidently given out, where divisor and dividend are both unknown.

Carlyle, *Sartor Resartus*

In a series of papers starting in 1928, Neyman and Pearson (NP hereafter) considered the following problem: given that there were a number of tests of significance that might be applied to a given problem how could one choose between them? The answer turned out to be related to Fisher's likelihood.

NP considered the extension of significance testing from being that of deciding whether or not to reject a null hypothesis to being that of choosing between a null and an alternative hypothesis. In a medical context the null hypothesis might be that a drug had no effect of blood pressure and the alternative that mean blood pressure was lowered, the distribution of blood pressure being otherwise unaffected. NP considered two types of error. An error of the first kind, committed by falsely rejecting the null hypothesis, and an error of the second kind committed by falsely rejecting the alternative hypothesis. In general, as the probability of one sort of error decreases the probability of the other increases.

Using this framework the following operational interpretation of significance tests could be given. If you have the habit of carrying out significance tests at (say) the 5% level, you will make a type I error in 5% of all cases when the null hypothesis is true. (You will obviously never make such an error when the null hypothesis is false.) NP then considered what would happen if, accepting a given type I error rate such as 0.05, one attempted to minimise the type II error rate or equivalently attempted to maximise one minus this rate, which they called the *power* of the test.

What NP showed in a famous 'lemma', was that an 'optimal' test (that is to say, most powerful for a given type I error rate) would satisfy a particular condition in terms of the likelihood.[24] One must consider all possible samples that might arise. A statistical test is a calculation based on such samples. The result of the calculation is either to accept or reject the null hypothesis. Hence, any given test can be characterised by saying which samples would lead to rejection and which to acceptance. For each possible sample the ratio of the likelihood under the alternative to the likelihood under the null should be calculated. This ratio provides a means of ranking the possible samples. Those with high values of the ratio give more support to the alternative hypothesis; those with low ratios give less support. What NP showed was that an optimal test is then one that satisfies the following condition: all the samples that would lead to rejection must have a higher ratio of the likelihood than all those which would lead to acceptance. The precise value of the ratio that defines the demarcation between acceptance and rejection must be chosen so that the type I error rate is of the requisite size *that is to say less than or equal to the tolerated type I error rate.*

Consider a coin tossing example. We wish to test the null hypothesis that the coin is fair against the alternative that the coin has a 0.2 probability of showing 'heads' and we are to toss the coin eight times and use a 5% level of significance. Consider a particular sequence of results, HTTTTHTT, where H = head and T = tail. The likelihood under the alternative hypothesis is obtained by multiplying the probability of a head (0.2) by that under a tail (0.8) by 0.8 again and so forth to obtain

$$0.2 \times 0.8 \times 0.8 \times 0.8 \times 0.8 \times 0.2 \times 0.8 \times 0.8 = 0.2^2 \times 0.8^6 = 0.0105.$$

A little thought makes it clear that this likelihood is the same for all sequences having the same number of heads and, if k is this number, is equal in general to $0.2^k 0.8^{(8-k)}$. On the other hand, the likelihood under the null hypothesis is $0.5^8 = (1/2)^8 = 1/256 = 0.0039$ for every sequence. The ratio of these two likelihoods is 2.68. In other words, the observed sequence is 2.68 times as likely under the alternative as under the null hypothesis. Table 4.1 calculates for every possible value of the number of heads k, the number of sequences s (obtained using Pascal's triangle or the formula), the probability under H_0 of obtaining that number of heads $p(k)$, the probability of

Table 4.1. *Probabilities and ratios of likelihoods for a coin-tossing example.*

k	s	p(k)	p(≤k)	λ
0	1	0.0039	0.0039	42.950
1	8	0.0312	0.0352	10.737
2	28	0.1094	0.1445	2.684
3	56	0.2188	0.3633	0.671
4	70	0.2734	0.6367	0.168
5	56	0.2188	0.8555	0.042
6	28	0.1094	0.9648	0.010
7	8	0.0312	0.9951	0.003
8	1	0.0039	1	0.001
Total	256	1.000		

obtaining that number or fewer of heads, $p(\leq k)$ and the ratio of likelihoods, λ.

What the NP lemma says is that if we want a test with a type I error rate of 0.0312 that is as powerful as possible, then we should reject the null hypothesis whenever one of the nine sequences corresponding to $k = 0$ or $k = 1$ is observed. If instead, for example, we rejected the null hypothesis whenever $k = 0$ or $k = 7$, we would have a test with the same type I error rate but this would not be as powerful against the given alternative. Equivalently, the test can be based upon the statistic which corresponds to the number of heads and if (in this case) this statistic has a value of 1 or less, the null hypothesis should be rejected. The NP lemma thus provides a way of choosing statistics, associated tests and rules of rejection based upon requirements of size and power. This seems to remove an unwelcome arbitrary element.

However, a number of problems remain. For example, we originally stated that we want a test of size 5%, not 3.12%. Then common sense seems to dictate that we should probably stick with the test we already have and accept the fact that it is conservative; that is to say accept that the type I error rate will be less than 5%. However, suppose that I adopt the following strategy. If $k = 1$ or less I reject the null hypothesis; if k is 3 or more I accept it. However if $k = 2$, I get my computer to generate a random number between nought and one.[25] If this random number is less than 0.135, I reject the null hypothesis. If the null hypothesis is true, the probability that we will reject it is now the probability that $k = 1$ or less plus the probability that it will equal 1 and that the random number will be less than 0.135. This total probability is $0.0352 + 0.135 \times 0.1094 = 0.05$ as required.

This manoeuvre seems absurd but the test now has the requisite type I error rate and greater power than it did before. If these are the only two requirements that drive the logic of the test this modification seems unobjectionable.

A further difficulty is that our unmodified test corresponds to accepting anything with a ratio of likelihoods of less than 10.74 in favour of the alternative hypothesis as being inadequate to support rejection of the null. However, if we increase the sample size whilst retaining the type I error rate it then turns out that the critical ratio gets smaller and smaller. Eventually, a situation can be reached where the null hypothesis will be rejected even though the ratio is less than unity (that is to say against the alternative).

Finally, consider the behaviour of a statistician who intends to carry out a series of hypothesis tests on similar questions and wishes to control the average type I error rate over the series (rather than for each test) whilst maximising the power. How should (s)he behave? It turns out that (s)he should carry out tests in such a way that the same critical ratio of likelihoods is maintained in the series of tests.[26]

These considerations tend to suggest that the common interpretation of the NP lemma, namely that the size and power requirements are fundamental and that the likelihood is the means of optimising power for a given size, are back to front. It is the likelihood requirement that is fundamental, and the power property is an incidental bonus. This subtle change in viewpoint requires no alteration to the NP lemma, which, being a mathematical object, is indeed 'correct'. It does, however, lead to a quite different attitude to hypothesis testing: one which places likelihood at the centre.

This is not a view, however, that Neyman himself would endorse. Neyman regarded the problem of inference as misstated. You could never know anything was true; you couldn't even have a belief in its truth. Its truth, or otherwise, was independent of you. All you could do was decide to behave as if it were true or false. The theory of hypothesis testing controlled your errors in so doing.

Karl Popper (1902–1994)

Karl Popper was born in Vienna of Jewish parents who had converted to Lutheranism before his birth.[27] His father was a Doctor of Law at the University of Vienna. After studying mathematics and physics at the University, during which time he was also apprenticed to a carpenter,

Popper worked as a secondary school teacher. In 1937 Popper, escaping Nazi persecution, emigrated to New Zealand where he had accepted a lectureship in Canterbury University College, Christchurch.

In 1945, after a helpful intervention by Hayek, Popper published his brilliant critical analysis of totalitarianism, *The Open Society and its Enemies*. This is one of the great books of the twentieth century and was to attract considerable criticism, not only for its attack on a then fashionable Marxism but for its even more hostile examination of Plato's *Republic*.

In 1946, again after the helpful intervention of Hayek, Popper was appointed a reader at the London School of Economics where he was to remain until his retirement. Popper is of interest to us here, however, for two reasons. First his propensity theory of probability and second his proposed falsificationist solution to Hume's theory of induction. The former theory claimed that probability was not a long-run relative frequency as (say) Neyman would maintain, nor a degree of belief as (say) Jeffreys would maintain, nor non-existent (as de Finetti would sometimes claim) but a tendency inherent in the properties of the system being studied: radioactive sources, dice, turbulent flow, and so forth. Whatever difficulties there may be with this theory, many statisticians behave as if this were true, especially when building statistical models.

Popper's approach to Hume's problem of induction was more radical. It was to point out that universal laws could not be proved but they could be disproved. Instead he suggested that the body of statements that made up scientific theories were precisely those that led to predictions that (if they did not occur) could prove the theories false. Science was thus a body of theories that were in principle falsifiable and it was the scientist's task to submit his/her theories to stringent tests in order that those that were false could be exposed as such.

Popper's approach is thus a philosophical system that appears superficially compatible with the NP system of hypothesis testing. In fact the NP approach as commonly applied is incompatible with Popper's system. The reason is that within the NP system the choice of null and alternative hypotheses is largely arbitrary. Consider bioequivalence testing. This is a field in which we try to show that two formulations of a pharmaceutical are the same by comparing their concentration time profiles in the blood, having given them to healthy volunteers who are then sampled frequently. It is usual to adopt the null hypothesis that the two formulations are different to a given degree (an amount that is just 'relevant') and 'disprove' this hypothesis in order to be able to assert the alternative hypothesis that they differ by no more than an irrelevant amount. The analogy would be to attempt to deal with Hume's problem of induction by declaring a scientific theory was false and then proving by contradiction that it was true. However, by this device all we could ever hope to do would be prove that it was not false in a given circumstance or set of circumstances, not that it was always true.

In fact, Popper's philosophical system is more like that of Fisher, who only allowed certain types of statement to fill the role of null hypothesis. However, there is another surprising and curious parallel and that is to de Finetti. Popper was a believer in objective and de Finetti in subjective knowledge but they had many views in common. (Politics excepted!) For example both admired Hume and both were critical of Plato (de Finetti much more so than Popper). Which of the two wrote this, 'The acquisition of a further piece of information, H – in other words experience, since experience is nothing more than the acquisition of further information – acts always and only in the way we have just described: suppressing the alternatives that turn out to be no longer possible . . .'?[28] This piece of pure falsificationism is in fact de Finetti and not Popper.

Where does this leave us?

If I knew the answer to this I would be in a position to issue a theory to rival those of de Finetti, Jeffreys, Neyman or Fisher. I am not. I finish instead with some personal remarks.

1. I consider that of all the various statistical theories of inference the single most impressive in the sense of apparently forming a coherent whole is de Finetti's.

2. However, I believe that de Finetti's theory is not enough. In particular it seems impossible to apply for any length of time and the scientist will not want to give up the possibility of saying 'back to the drawing board', a statement that the theory forbids.

3. I speculate that a fuller theory will have to incorporate elements of both the falsificationist view of Popper and the subjective probability system of de Finetti.[29]

4. In the meantime the practising statistician can do no better than follow George Barnard's injunction to be familiar with the four major systems of statistical inference; namely; Fisher's, Neyman's and Pearson's, Jeffreys's and de Finetti's.[30]

Finally I offer this koan by way of encouraging insight which, if it is not quite Zen, is at least pure Senn.

The jealous husband's dilemma

The jealous husband fears that his wife is unfaithful and determines to try to set his mind at ease. He hires a private detective to investigate her. Several weeks and large sums of money later, the detective issues his report. He has followed the wife for weeks, investigated her phone calls and observed her every movement. In an extensive report he explains that there is no evidence whatsoever that she is having an affair.

The husband is much relieved. His prior doubt has been changed into posterior belief. He goes to bed with a light heart for the first time in months. At three o' clock in the morning he wakes with a frightening thought . . . suppose his wife is having an affair with the detective?

5

Sex and the single patient

He wanted a record of the effect of race, occupation, and a dozen other factors upon the disease rate.

Sinclair Lewis, Arrowsmith

Splitters and poolers

The world can be divided into those who split and those who pool. For the former, the devil is in the detail. There is no point in talking about the effect of a given treatment on patients in general. Patients do not arrive 'in general' at the surgery door, they arrive in particular and it is personal treatment they seek (or at least, this is generally the case). For the latter, what is applicable to one is applicable to one and all. The world is awash with chance and contingency. Only by repeated study and by averaging can we hope to make any sense of it at all.

On the whole, physicians are splitters and statisticians are poolers. Being a statistician I can make that sort of statement. If I were a physician, I would have difficulty in saying anything about it at all.

In fact, intermediate positions are possible, and certain statistical approaches, most notably the Bayesian one, address this explicitly. The Bayesian approach would be to use one's prior belief that apparently similar things often behave in fairly similar ways. It is a matter of reasonable belief, for example, that the effect of a treatment is unlikely to be very different when applied to Roman Catholics then when applied to Anglicans. It may differ rather more in its effects on men and women, although even here similarity may be expected. For example, we should be extremely surprised to find that a treatment that cured athlete's foot in men would kill women similarly afflicted.

Nevertheless, we know that there can be important differences. For example, isoniazid, a drug used to treat tuberculosis, is acetylised slowly by some individuals, a condition that could lead to overdosing and toxicity. The distribution of slow acetylisers is different among different ethnic groups, being more common amongst Caucasians than amongst Orientals.[1] Furthermore, such differences do not need to be genetic. Grapefruit juice interferes with the elimination of several drugs including ciclosporin, used in transplantation surgery, and carbamazapine, used in epilepsy. With some drugs the grapefruit effect can lead to a three-fold increase in the concentration of the drug in the blood with obvious potential for side-effects.[2] Since consumption of grapefruit juice is likely to vary from culture to culture, we here have a possible apparent justification for looking at our trial results cross-classified by social class, country, ethnicity, sex and so forth.

With such potential variety, how are we to make progress at all in discovering the effects of treatment? This is one of the sore puzzles facing the medical statistician and in this chapter we consider the issues. But before considering the statistics we consider the politics, because if this has become a hot topic, it is politicians who have provided the heat.

Doctors become patients

The Physicians' Health Study was bold and imaginative. The originators wished to investigate the effect of aspirin in a dose of 325 milligrams per day on cardiovascular mortality and of β-carotene 50 milligrams per day on cancer. To do this they employed a so-called factorial design. Subjects were split into four groups as shown in Table 5.1.

Table 5.1. *Groups in the Physicians' Health Study.*

		β-Carotene	
		No	Yes
	No	Placebo to aspirin plus placebo to β-carotene	Placebo to aspirin plus β-carotene
Aspirin			
	Yes	Aspirin plus placebo to β-carotene	Aspirin plus β-carotene

Factorial designs are a type of study pioneered in connection with agricultural experiments by the Rothamsted school of statistics founded by R. A. Fisher but are perhaps now more closely associated with the name of his chief disciple Frank Yates than with the master himself. In the statistician's argot, aspirin and β-carotene are *factors* and presence ('yes') and absence ('no') are *levels*. Here each of the two factors has two levels and the study is then referred to as a 2×2 factorial experiment. (Had the trial used 'no', 'low' and 'high' doses of aspirin, this factor would then have had three levels.)

The beauty of a factorial experiment is that not only do you get two or more (depending on the number of factors) experiments for the price of one, but you can also look at interactions between factors. In this example you could study whether the effect of aspirin and β-carotene together is more or less than the sum of their effects taken alone. However, this experiment is not quite a factorial experiment in the classical sense since that would study the effect of the factors on the same outcome variable. (Typically, in the agricultural context one would study the effect on yield.) In the Physicians' Health Study, however, the effects of aspirin and β-carotene are being studied on different outcomes, cardiovascular mortality and cancer, and their interaction was not really of interest.

Factorial designs are rarely used in clinical trials, but this relatively unusual feature was not the main interest of the study. The principle interest of this trial was that the subjects were, '22 071 U.S. male physicians between the ages of 40–84 years'.[3] The treatments were prophylactic so that the subjects were healthy individuals rather than patients. Using physicians as the subjects made it possible to achieve high compliance. The trial was conducted entirely by post and was extremely cost-effective. Although initiated in the mid 1980s, the subjects in the trial are still being followed up. However, results to date suggest that that although β-carotene does not prevent cancer, aspirin is effective in preventing heart disease.

The raucous caucus

Or is it? That was spoken like a pooler. What would the splitters say? After all, the subjects in the study were all men. Can the results be applied to women? This was indeed the question that was posed by various female politicians in the US. Outraged by the fact the women had not been included in the Physicians' Health Study, the 'Women's Congressional

Caucus', headed by Patricia Schroeder, a Democrat Representative for Colorado, and Barbara Mikulski, a Democrat Senator for Maryland, insisted that trials funded by the National Institutes of Health (NIH) had to be organised in such a way as to ensure adequate representation of women. As Senator Mikulski later put it when addressing the US Senate in October 1992, 'Men and women stood by the congressional women 2 years ago. On the day when we women marched up the steps of the NIH asking to be included in medical studies and cures for repugnant diseases . . . We knew what the statistics were for men – but no one had ever bothered to look at the fact that women get heart disease too.'[4]

As it turned out the claimed neglect was not true but it was widely believed at the time. In a very careful examination of the literature on clinical trials, Curtis Meinert and co-workers, in a paper published in 2000, were able to show that women were not being ignored by trialists.[5] In 100 455 trials published in US journals 55% involved men and women, 12% involved men only, 11% involved women only and in 21% the policy could not be determined from the description. For 724 trials published in five leading journals, the numbers of men and women included were 355 624 and 550 734 respectively. Meinert et al. found no evidence that prior to the action from the 'Women's Caucus', women had been under-represented in clinical trials.

But what about the dollar picture? The NIH Advisory Committee on Women's Health Issues had prepared a report in 1989. This showed that expenditure on diseases or condition specifically related to women as a percentage of total NIH expenditure was 12% and 14% for the fiscal years 1986 and 1987. This was misunderstood by some to imply that the 88% and 86% was spent on men. In fact, much of the rest of the money was being spent on issues relevant to both males and females and very little of it was spent on men alone. As Meinert et al. showed, from 1988 to 1998 the yearly ratio of expenditure females to men was never less than 1.8 (1991) and was as high as 2.8 (1996).

And finally, what about health itself. Do women do worse than men? Figure 5.1 shows life-expectancy for both sexes averaged over all races for the USA from 1940 to 1990. It shows a fact that was known to John Arbuthnot at the beginning of the eighteenth century. Whatever the vicissitudes either sex faces from 'repugnant diseases', to use Senator Mikulski's phrase, women live longer on average than men. It seems that in terms of one rather important outcome of health, life, women are not an underprivileged underclass. This is not say that underprivileged classes

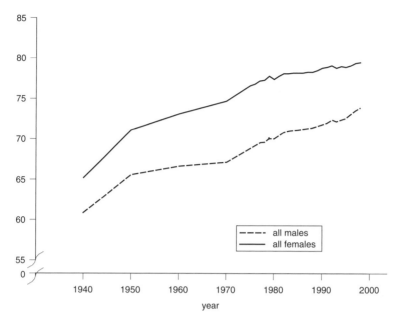

Figure 5.1 Life expectancy 1940, 1950, 1960, 1970 and 1975–1998 by sex for all races in the USA. Source: *National Vital Statistics Reports*, 2000; **48** (11): 24 July.

do not exist. For example the life-expectancy of whites in the USA is considerably more than that of blacks. In fact so strong is this disparity that the life expectancy of black women is scarcely more than that of white men.

So concerned were the US politicians, however, about the supposed bias against women that the 103rd Congress devoted valuable time to debate and pass legislation to require the director of NIH to ensure that trials be 'designed and carried out in a manner sufficient to provide for a valid analysis of whether the variables being studied in the trial affect women or members of minority subgroups, as the case may be differently than other subjects in the trial'.[6] As we shall see however, this requirement, if fulfilled, would be disastrous for the conduct of clinical trials.

Power to the people

In designing a clinical trial some attention is usually paid to ensure that the trial has adequate 'power'. This is a technical term associated in particular with the Neyman–Pearson theory of testing for hypotheses and it was covered in Chapter 4. The way it works in the pharmaceutical industry is as follows. The medical statistician assigned to help design the trial is given a licence to drive the physician crazy by pestering him or her for 'the clinically relevant difference'. This mysterious quantity is needed to decide how many patients to assign to the trial. The more patients that are assigned, the greater the probability that the 'signal' from a given treatment effect, to use an analogy from engineering, will be detectable against the background 'noise' of random variation and will allow one to conclude that the treatment works. This does not happen because increasing the number of patients increases the signal. It is rather that it reduces the level of background noise. As our old friend the Marquis de Laplace put it, 'The phenomena of nature are most often enveloped by so many strange circumstances, and so great a number of disturbing causes mix their influence, that it is very difficult to recognise them. We may arrive at them only by multiplying the observations or the experiences, so that the strange effects finally destroy reciprocally each other.'[7]

This reciprocal destruction of strange effects obeys an inverse square root law so that, other things being equal, to reduce the noise by a half you have to quadruple the sample size. What you are aiming for in the trial is a given signal-to-noise ratio, to use the engineering analogy again. The problem, however, is that you do not know what the strength of the signal is, this being the unknown treatment effect. This is where the clinically relevant difference comes into its own. It is sometimes described as the difference you would not like to miss. When I worked in the pharmaceutical industry I used to encourage my colleagues to think about it as follows. 'If the trial is negative, it is quite likely that this project will be cancelled. This means that this drug will *never* be studied again. It will be lost to Mankind *forever*. Bearing in mind that there are other drugs waiting to be studied, what is the maximum level of effect at which we would be able to tolerate the loss of such a drug?'

Once the clinically relevant difference has been determined and a type I error rate of the test to be used for comparing treatment groups has been established, a target power is used to determine the size of the trial. The *type I error rate* is the probability with which the null hypothesis that the treatment effect (comparing experimental treatment to control) is zero will be rejected if it is true. The *power* of the test is then the probability with which the null hypothesis will be rejected if it is false and if the clinically relevant difference obtains. The type I error rate and the power together determine the signal-to-noise ratio that it is necessary to achieve.

For example, using the common standard of a type I error rate of 2.5% and a power of 80%, it is necessary to achieve a signal-to-noise ratio of 2.8.

Now consider a concrete example. Suppose that we have determined in a placebo-controlled trial in asthma that the clinically relevant difference in terms of forced expiratory volume in one second (FEV_1) is 280 ml. That is to say, we should not like to miss any drug that produced more than 280 ml bronchodilation compared to placebo. The statistician's 'noise' measure, the measurement of variability used, is called the *standard error*. We thus require to design a trial for which the ratio of clinically relevant difference to standard error is 2.8. In other words we need a standard error of 280 ml/2.8 = 100 ml. Note that the standard error is measured in the same units as the clinically relevant difference.

It turns out that the standard error depends on four things: first, the design of the experiment; second, the type of analysis employed; third, the number of patients studied; and finally the variability of the raw data. Statisticians commonly use two measures to describe such variability in the data. The first, the standard deviation for which the symbol σ (a lower case Greek sigma) is commonly used, is measured on the same scale as the data themselves. (In ml of FEV_1 in this example.) The second, the variance, is simply the square of the standard deviation, σ^2. This squared scale is often useful for performing calculations.

On the assumption that a little maths, if occasionally exhausting, is nevertheless good exercise, we shall try to justify some formulae that we are going to use in discussing the representation of women in clinical trials. The reader who disagrees should 'fast-forward' three sections.

The mental traveller*

I traveld thro' a Land of Men
A Land of Men & Women too

William Blake, The Mental Traveller

We divert for a while to consider the statistician's measures of variability, the variance and standard deviation. To help us understand this, consider a simple question in geography and geometry. An explorer in a flat desert walks three miles west and then four miles north. How far away is she from her starting point? We shall ignore any nice problems to do with the Earth's curvature in answering this and assume, instead, that we can treat this as a straightforward problem in two-dimensional Euclidean geometry.

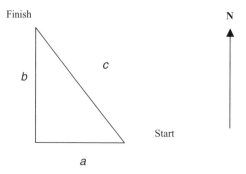

To solve this problem we can use one of the most famous theorems in all mathematics, that of Pythagoras. The imaginary line joining the point of arrival to the point of departure of our explorer completes a triangle. Because she walked north, having first walked west this is a right triangle and the distance we seek is that of the hypotenuse, the other two being given. Pythagoras's theorem says that the square on the hypotenuse is equal to the sum of the squares on the other two sides. We thus calculate 3 miles² + 4 miles² = 9 square miles plus 16 square miles = 25 square miles. The square on the hypotenuse is thus 25 square miles, from which it follows that the hypotenuse is 5 miles. Our explorer is five miles from her starting point.

The general algebraic rule that reflects Pythagoras's theorem, and which we can use, is as follows. If someone walks a distance a and then turns at right angles and walks a further distance b they are now a distance c from their starting point, where c satisfies the equation

$$c^2 = a^2 + b^2. \tag{5.1}$$

Now suppose that although our explorer had walked three miles west as before, she had then continued on her journey by walking 4 miles northwest. The generalisation of Pythagoras's theorem to cover cases where the triangle is not a right angle can be expressed algebraically in terms of the so-called *cosine law*, as

$$c^2 = a^2 + b^2 - 2ab \cos C, \tag{5.2}$$

where C is the angle opposite to side c and $\cos C$ is the cosine of this angle. In the case of our original example, we had a right-angled triangle so that C was 90°. $\cos 90°$ is 0 so that Pythagoras's theorem can be seen as a special case of the cosine law corresponding to the angle between the two sides being 90°.

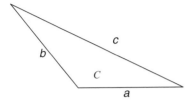

In the case of our explorer, the angle C is $90° + 45° = 135°$ and $\cos C = \cos 135°$ which equals $-1/\sqrt{2} \approx -0.707$. Thus we calculate

$$c^2 = 3 \text{ miles}^2 + 4 \text{ miles}^2 - 2 \times 3 \text{ miles} \times 4 \text{ miles} \times -0.707$$
$$c^2 = (9 + 16 + 17.0) \text{ miles}^2 = 41.968 \text{ miles}^2$$
$$c = 6.5 \text{ miles}.$$

By this time the reader will be asking what the point is of this diversion. The answer is that variability in statistics obeys analogous rules to these distance rules. Suppose that we have two measurements (which we denote using symbols X_1 and X_2 respectively). We do not take these measurements perfectly but suppose that they may have some error attached to them so that they would vary from occasion to occasion. Assume, further, that they can vary randomly and *independently*, which is to say that what happens in measuring the one has no influence on the measurement of the other. The unknown true value of the first measurement is μ_1 and the unknown true value of the second is μ_2 and the observed values X_1 and X_2 will be either greater or less than these true values with no bias in either direction. The variability with which the observed measurements will differ from these true values is described by standard deviations σ_1 and σ_2 respectively. Now suppose that we decide to add some multiple of the one, say a, to some multiple of the other, say b. In general we may say we calculate $Y = aX_1 + bX_2$. What, using the vocabulary of statistics, would we *expect* this value to be, which is to say, what should it be on average? The answer is, quite trivially, that we expect it to be $a\mu_1 + b\mu_2$.

Now suppose that we ask a more difficult question. Since X_1 and X_2 are measurements that can vary randomly and Y is calculated from these quantities, Y must also vary randomly. What is its standard deviation? If we call the standard deviation of Y, σ_Y, so that its variance is σ_Y^2, it turns out that we have the following Pythagorean rule for its variance

$$\sigma_Y^2 = a^2\sigma_1^2 + b^2\sigma_2^2. \tag{5.3}$$

In the special case where the variance of X_1 is the same as the variance of X_2 and is equal to σ_2 (say), we can write

$$\sigma_Y^2 = a^2\sigma^2 + b^2\sigma^2$$
$$\sigma_Y^2/\sigma^2 = a^2 + b^2$$
$$c^2 = a^2 + b^2,$$

where c is the ratio of the standard deviation of Y to the standard deviation of an original measurement. But this is of the same form as Pythagoras's formula (5.1).

Just as we required a more general formula when our explorer did not move at right angles, so a more general formula is needed for the variance of Y when X_1 and X_2 are not independent as might be the case say if some common cause was effecting our two measurements. Just as we needed a further trigonometric concept, that of the cosine for this case, so we need a further statistical concept, that of the *covariance* to cover the case where the measurements are not independent. Our formula now becomes

$$\sigma_Y^2 = a^2\sigma_1^2 + b^2\sigma_2^2 + 2ab\,\mathrm{cov}_{12} \tag{5.4}$$

where cov_{12} is the covariance of X_1 and X_2.

When we take again the case where X_1 and X_2 have the same variance, σ^2, then we may write

$$\sigma_Y^2/\sigma^2 = a^2 + b^2 = 2ab\,\mathrm{cov}_{12}/\sigma^2$$
$$c^2 = a^2 + b^2 = 2ab\rho, \tag{5.5}$$

where $\rho = \mathrm{cov}_{12}/\sigma^2$ (in this case) is a quantity called the *correlation coefficient*, first named by Francis Galton and developed extensively by Karl Pearson. Just like the cosine of an angle, the correlation coefficient lies between -1 and $+1$.

If (5.5) is compared to (5.2) it will be seen to be the same if $\cos C$ is replaced by $-\rho$. In fact, the correlation coefficient is positive if X_1 and X_2 tend to vary sympathetically, that is to say, if X_2 tends to be above its true value when X_1 is above its true value. On the other hand, the correlation is negative if the variables vary antithetically, which is to say that when one is higher than expected, the other tends to be lower than expected. The analogy, however, to sympathetic variation for our desert traveller is that the second direction should be closer to the first than the neutral case of walking at right angles. This was, indeed, the case in the second example when she walked north-west having first walked west. The cosine was negative and this is, of course, true for all angles in the range 90°–270° which means that we can regard the correlation coefficient as being analogous to the negative of the cosine in which case (5.5) will be seen to be perfectly analogous to (5.2).

Variation on a theme*

Pythagoras's theorem generalises to many dimensions. It is rather difficult to imagine travel in more than three so let us consider a three-dimensional example. Suppose, returning to our explorer's original journey, that having travelled 3 miles west and 4 miles north she now levitates vertically 12 miles into the air. How far will she be from her starting point? To answer this we can use Pythagoras's theorem again. She was 5 miles away from her starting point when she levitated and she is now 12 miles high. These are two sides of a further right-angled triangle the hypotenuse of which is the line whose length we seek. The square of this is equal to 5 miles^2 + 12 miles^2 = 25 miles^2 + 144 miles^2 = 169, from which it follows that the distance we seek is 13 miles. (Since the square of 13 is 169.)

Obviously the solution could also be obtained by adding the three squares of the distances together. So, changing our notation slightly, and considering travel in n dimensions we have,

$$h^2 = d_1^2 + d_2^2 + \cdots d_n^2, \tag{5.6}$$

where h is our generalised hypotenuse and $d_1, d_2 \cdots d_n$, are the sides of our n-dimensional triangle.

Now suppose, to return to statistics and variation, that we construct a weighted sum of n measurements. That is to say we take the first measurement X_1 (say) and multiply it by some constant k_1 (say) and then take the next measurement X_2 and multiply that by k_2 and so forth up to X_n and k_n and then add these n products together. Why we should choose to do such a strange thing will become clear shortly. The analogous equation to (5.6) for a variance of the sum of n independent measurements, each of which has been multiplied by some known quantity, is

$$V = k_1^2 \sigma_1^2 + k_2^2 \sigma_2^2 + \cdots + k_n^2 \sigma_n^2. \tag{5.7}$$

If the variance of each of these measurements is the same, say σ^2, then (5.7) reduces to

$$V = k_1^2\sigma^2 + k_2^2\sigma^2 + \cdots + k_n^2\sigma^2 = \sigma^2\left(k_1^2 + k_2^2 + \cdots k_n^2\right). \tag{5.8}$$

Now suppose that we have n patients in a particular treatment group in a clinical trial and we measure the outcome, say FEV_1, at the end of the trial for each of these patients. Each measurement can be regarded as a measurement on the effect of the treatment. Suppose we wish to calculate the average FEV_1 for the group as a whole. How reliable is this average?

Well, of course, that depends on many things. The patients we have chosen may be a rather unrepresentative bunch and the measurements may therefore be rather biased. The clinical trial will, in fact, deal with this bias element in a strikingly simple way and for the moment we shall not consider it. Instead we shall consider what the random variation in our result will be.

Suppose we calculate the mean result for these patients. (On average, when statisticians say mean, they mean average.) We can calculate this by dividing each of the n measurements and adding them. We can thus write

$$\overline{X} = X_1/n + X_2/n + \cdots X_n/n. \tag{5.9}$$

The result for one patient should not (usually) affect that for another so that we can reasonably regard the various X values as independent. Making the further assumption that variability is constant, we can then use (5.8) to obtain the variance of the mean, $\overline{X}$. Note that the multiplier for each X is $1/n$, this means that the multiplier for the variance terms is $1/n^2$. We thus write:

$$\mathrm{var}(\overline{X}) = \sigma^2\left(1/n^2 + 1/n^2 \cdots 1/n^2\right) = \sigma^2 n/n^2 = \sigma^2/n, \tag{5.10}$$

where, because we have n terms $1/n^2$, we have been able to cancel a term in n to obtain σ^2/n.

We have thus obtained a measure of the reliability of the mean of n observations. However, our measure is a variance and is in squared units. It is more useful, ultimately, to have a measurement that is on the same scale as the mean itself and so we take the square root of the variance. This is a sort of standard deviation of the mean but the linguistic convention is to refer to this as a *standard error*. Thus we have $SE(\overline{X}) = \sigma/\sqrt{n}$.

Returning to trials (and tribulations)*

When we wish to compare two treatments in a clinical trial then the precision with which we can measure each of them turns out to be important. Take the simplest case, where we have a parallel group trial in which patients are allocated at random to either the experimental treatment or control, with n_t and n_c patients in the respective groups. Suppose we perform the simplest of all analyses in which we subtract the mean result from one group from the mean in the other. Suppose that we call this 'statistic', this difference in means, D. It has been calculated as $D = \overline{X}_t - \overline{X}_c$. However both $\overline{X}_t$, the mean in the treatment group, and $\overline{X}_c$, the mean in the control group, are random variables, which is to say their values may vary. Furthermore D is a statistic of the form $Y = aX_1 + bX_2$ with $X_1 = \overline{X}_t$, $X_2 = \overline{X}_c$, $a = 1$ and $b = -1$. Furthermore, $\overline{X}_t$ and $\overline{X}_c$ are independent and, if we assume that the original observations have a common variance σ^2, have variances σ^2/n_t and σ^2/n_c respectively. Hence since $a^2 = 1$ and $b^2 = 1$, application of (5.3) yields $\text{var}(D) = \sigma^2(1/n_t + 1/n_c)$ from which we obtain the following formula for the standard error, SE:

$$\text{SE} = \sigma \sqrt{\frac{1}{n_t} + \frac{1}{n_c}}. \tag{5.11}$$

Here n_t is the number of patients in the treatment group and n_c is the number in the control group.

This apparently simple formula has a number of consequences. For example, other things being equal, if we increase the number of patients in either group, n_t or n_c, then the standard error will reduce. However, given a total number of patients N, where N is therefore the sum of n_t and n_c, then it will pay us to allocate patients as equally as possible. Under such circumstances we have $n_t = n_c = N/2$ and substituting in (5.11) we obtain the following formula for the minimum SE, $\text{SE}_{\min}$:

$$\text{SE}_{\min} = \sigma \sqrt{\frac{4}{N}}. \tag{5.12}$$

A bout de souffle

Return to our example. The clinically relevant difference was 280 ml and we established that in order to have 80% power to detect this difference given a type I error rate of 5% we had to achieve a standard error of 100 ml.

Suppose that the standard deviation, σ, is 400 ml, then it will be seen if this, together with the value for N of 64, is substituted in (5.12) a result of 100 ml obtains. Hence, we need 64 patients for the trial.

Or do we? This was before the Women's Caucus struck their blow for equality and against repugnant diseases. Let us remind ourselves of the legislation. Trials must be 'designed and carried out in a manner sufficient to provide for a valid analysis of whether the variables being studied in the trial affect women or members of minority subgroups, as the case may be differently than other subjects in the trial'. How would we establish this? Up to now we have been considering designing the trial to show that the treatment works at all. Now we have to show whether it works differently in women, for example, than in men. We can do this by calculating a treatment effect for men, the difference between the two treatments for men alone, and then doing the same for women and finally by comparing these two difference. Let us call the first difference D_m and the second D_w, and the difference between the two D_{sex}. This sort of double difference is called the 'interactive effect' by statisticians. If it can be shown to be 'significant' then (putting aside any objections to significance tests as aids to reasoning) there is a sex-by-treatment interaction.

Now suppose that we have N patients in general and that we use the allocation of sexes and treatment for this trial, which for a given number of patients will give the most precise answer. This requires N/4 patients on each of the four groups: males on treatment and control and females on treatment and control. If we now calculate the standard error for D_m, the difference between treatment and control for males, we now have to substitute N/4 for n_t and n_c in (5.11) to obtain, as an alternative to (5.12)

$$SE_m = \sigma\sqrt{\frac{8}{N}}. \tag{5.13}$$

We thus now appear to need twice as many patients to achieve the same precision. However, matters are worse than this. We now have to compare D_m to D_f and this requires us to calculate the standard error of the double difference D_{sex}. We thus have to use our Pythagorean rule again of squaring and adding. In other words we have to add two variances, each of which is the square of (5.13), and then take the square root to obtain

$$SE_{sex} = \sigma\sqrt{\frac{16}{N}}. \tag{5.14}$$

Thus, our trial that previously required 64 patients now requires 256.

All this of course is on the assumption that the clinically relevant difference for the effect of treatment between the sexes is not smaller than that for the treatment as a whole. It clearly cannot be larger. For example, we said that 280 ml was the clinically relevant difference overall. We could hardly accept (say) a clinically relevant difference for the interaction of 300 ml, since this could occur if the treatment improved FEV_1 by 280 ml for men and made it worse by 20 ml for women. In practice it could be argued that the clinically relevant difference for the interactive effect ought to be less than 280 ml and this, of course, would push the sample size up still further.

But we are still not at an end with the difficulties. We have to do this examination not just for women but also for other demographic subgroups many of which are minorities. In any case for many diseases men and women are very unequally represented. For example, osteoporosis is much more likely to affect women whereas lung cancer is more common in men. The formulae that we have been using assume the optimal allocation of patients from the point of view of minimising the standard error for the total number of patients in the trial. As already explained, this requires equal numbers in each subgroup. However, if the disease is unequally represented in the demographic subgroups in the population, this requires us to sample unequally from the various strata. In a trial in lung cancer, we should have recruited our quota of male subjects long before the quota of females was reached. This means that the effect on recruitment time will be to more than quadruple it.

The alternative approach of accepting unequal numbers in each subgroup means that to achieve the same precision the trial size will have to more than quadruple. Either way, the quadrupling is an underestimate of the effect on trial times. Although the budget for it will not have quadrupled, since there are some common overheads, it will have increased substantially and this will reduce the funding available elsewhere for fighting those repugnant diseases. As the saying goes, 'parallel trials meet at infinity but this is more patients than you can afford'.

Bias binding

There is a side issue that needs to picked up here. We said earlier that clinical trials do not (in general) succeed in recruiting representative patients. This will be true, even if we take care to examine the differences between subgroups in the way that the US Congress required. In fact, this will be especially true if we look at sex (or race) by treatment interaction since we are likely, in order to have enough power, to over-recruit from minority groups. In any case, simply because we have specified so many whites, so many blacks, so many males, so many females, so many white males, and so forth does not mean that the sample is representative. Take the case of the Physicians' Health Study; even if it had included women there would have been no lawyers – and no politicians for that matter.

As regards one of the purposes of a clinical trial, which is to investigate whether the treatment *can* work, this does not matter. This is because we can still compare like with like. Again consider the Physicians' Health Study. Whatever explanations there might be for the finding that aspirin has a beneficial effect on cardiovascular mortality, this result cannot be explained away by saying that the trial recruited men only.

The situation is quite different if we run a trial in which men and women are represented but all the women receive aspirin and all the men receive placebo. A difference in mortality between the two treatment groups would also be a difference in mortality between the sexes and we would have difficulty deciding which was responsible.

This sort of bias is dealt with very effectively by the randomised clinical trial. Like is compared with like and although this like may not be typical it is at least fair. Blocking and statistical modelling (effectively a form of matching) deals with the presence of known confounding variables. (Known to epidemiologists as 'confounders'). Randomisation deals with hidden confounders.

Fair sex

So what have trialists done? Have they increased the size of their trials by a factor of at least four and the time to recruit patients by the same? No. Of course they haven't. They have decided to act in the interests of all women and men and blacks and whites, in short, of people. Attempts to put into practice the letter of the law that Congress passed would have been doomed to failure. The main problems with looking for effective cures are first that there aren't enough resources, second the cures usually make modest gains in health and, therefore, third we want to keep on looking. There is no point searching over the same piece of ground in yet finer detail when there is so much to explore.

Nobody wants trials that take four times as long to complete. Life is too short and all of us are dying. And we don't want politicians to make these stupid decisions on our behalf. If the trialists have found a treatment that increases survival in lung cancer but most of the patients have been men, very few women with lung cancer want to see the trials continue.

So what is the net result? A very gratifying tokenism develops. Trialists (quite sensibly) run trials the way they always have done, making if necessary a few placatory noises to grant-making bodies. Politicians go about their business, safe in the knowledge that they have struck a blow against sexism in science. (Of course a cynic might say that they have simply made it easier to use women's bodies to develop drugs for men.) And sexual politics and the clinical trial? For some reason, I am reminded of Ambrose Bierce's definition of a platitude; 'A jelly-fish withering on the shore of the sea of thought'.

6

A hale view of pills (and other matters)

I only treat illnesses that don't exist: that way if I can't cure them, there's no harm done.

Norton Juster, *The Phantom Tollbooth*

The post hoc, passed hack fallacy

The institution in which I profess statistics is UCL.[1] (Initially it was called University College London but now it is called initially. This has something to with branding, apparently.) My department is Statistical Science, the oldest such department in the world, and we are very proud of it. Indeed, it will not have escaped the attention of the attentive reader, that the typical founding father of statistics studied mathematics at Cambridge and then went on to lecture in statistics at UCL. This combination can easily be explained by observing that only Cambridge is good enough for statistics but statistics is not quite good enough for Cambridge.[2]

Returning to UCL, like other departments of statistics throughout Britain and indeed like departments in other disciplines, we have to document our excellence every five years. This is an extremely embarrassing business in which normally shy and retiring dons with no desire whatsoever for self-aggrandisement are forced by cruel and bitter economic and political exigency to list all their publications and public lectures for the 'Research Assessment Exercise'. Ah, cruel new world. Whatever happened to scholarship?

The statistics panel required us to submit our four best publications to be assessed. It is this that helped the assessors to determine whether we deserved the accolade of a five rating or the ignominy of a one. We were also expected to submit a list of all relevant publications. I did not, for the last quinquennial review, include my letter on the subject of Viagra to the street magazine, *The Big Issue*, despite the fact that it was the 'Star Letter' that week. This is not because the point it makes is not true but simply that it is so obvious that almost any human being who is not a journalist can understand it. The point is that just because one event sometimes follows another it does not follow that the following event is caused by that by which it is preceded. That this fallacy does, in fact, regularly get past your average journalist entitles it to a name: *the post hoc, passed hack fallacy*.[3]

Hacks and facts

I said, 'but I do know when I saw Guernsey beat Jersey in the Muratti, it was the best side won.' He said, 'How about when Jersey beat Guernsey?' 'Oh, that was just luck, I said.'

GB Edwards, *The Book of Ebenezer Le Page*

The letter I wrote was in response to the article: 'Viagra special report. Sex drug linked to 31 deaths in one year'. It turned out that a number of people who have taken Viagra are now dead. 'It was marketed as the wonder cure for impotence. But a year after being licensed in Britain, 31 users have died. Who is to blame?'[4] Who indeed? I blame it on the fact that more and more people going into journalism seem to have graduated in 'media studies'.

This is what I wrote.

Journalistic impotence

Viagra may be poison for all I know but your article 'Viagra: one year 31 deaths' (*Big Issue* **350**) left me not one jot the wiser on this subject. It would not surprise me to learn that several hundred former readers of the *Big Issue* are now dead. The Reaper does have this way with humans given enough of them and enough time to act. Perhaps you should withdraw the *Issue* from the streets pending an investigation. What was missing from your article was an estimate of the total exposure to Viagra and whether the number of deaths in the population of Viagra users was greater than expected given their numbers, their age and the time they were taking the drug.

If only they could invent a drug that would cure journalistic impotence and permit hacks to have some meaningful intercourse with science. Now there would be a medical breakthrough.[5]

Of course, they changed the title of my letter. It appeared as 'Viagra is a Big Flop' but this is usual. Sub-editors will rarely improve your grammar but will always change the titles of, 'letters to the editor'. It is one of the ways that they know they are needed. Nevertheless, to the credit of *The Big Issue*, the letter was otherwise uncensored.

Doomsbury

As everybody knows, John Maynard Keynes famously remarked, 'in the long run we are all dead'.[6] This is often the only thing that that somebody will know about Keynes except, perhaps, that he was a member of the Bloomsbury Set and hence inherently interesting, important and almost certainly sexually innovative and/or immoral depending on perspective. Certainly the long run has long since overtaken the Bloomsbury Set, who are all dead. Karl Marx famously spent a lot of time in Bloomsbury but this was in the reading room of the British Museum and not in its salons. In any case, his run ended in the year that JMK was born, which was far too early to appreciate that history repeats itself not only as tragedy and then as farce[7] but also, in the case of Bloomsbury, frequently in the Sunday papers. When I was a student of economics and statistics in the early seventies, an era before monetarism swept the world, Keynes was regarded as the greatest of all economists by all those who were actually thinking about economics rather than merely observing the inevitable historical working-out of dialectic materialism. What was not mentioned to us students was that he had also written an important treatise on probability. In fact, it was really as a response to this treatise that Frank Ramsey (whom we encountered in Chapter 4) wrote his own even more important essay on probability, now regarded as a precocious precursor of the neo-Bayesian era.

However, it is not for his revolutionary theories on general equilibrium and employment, nor even for his views on probability that Keynes is important to us here. It is precisely his views on death and the long run that are important. There would be a great improvement in the reporting of scientific and health matters in the newspapers if journalists could not only quote Keynes's most famous remark (as we all can) but actually understood what it meant. It means quite simply that in the long run we are all dead. Keynes's purpose, of course, was to point to the folly of allowing the long run to solve our economic problems. However, his great axiom, when supported by another couple, namely 'eventually the long run arrives', and 'some of us have been running quite a while', leads to the following very simple theorem. As the product of persons studied and the time they are studied increases then, under any conditions whatsoever, some of them will die *almost surely*.[8] A corollary of this important theorem is that when a large group of people have been studied for some time and it is found that some of them have died it does not necessarily follow that they have, as a group, been subject to unusually dangerous forces.

I apologise to the general reader for this unnecessarily laboured and obvious discussion. This particular section has been for the benefit of journalists and graduates of media studies, who may now skip the rest of this chapter as being too demanding, albeit not as sensational as that which famously dealt with the fall of the rupee.[9]

Comparisons after the fact

So how does one decide if the number of deaths, or adverse events, or other outcomes is greater than one might expect for a given group of individuals? One approach we have already encountered is that of the randomised controlled clinical trial. We study under identical conditions at the same time a control group not given the 'treatment' under consideration. This is not always practical. In particular, when reacting to news of the sort that made *The Big Issue* after it has broken, it is too late to do this. Instead we may have to use a second-best approach of constructing a similar group from other, perhaps historical, material.

We shall illustrate this approach with the help of one of the most curious figures in the statisco-historical menagerie.

Francis Galton (1822–1911)

Francis Galton[10] and Charles Darwin shared, in Erasmus Darwin, a famous grandfather. However Charles's father and Francis's mother were only half siblings, since Charles's father was the son of Erasmus's first wife, Mary Howard, whereas Francis's mother was the son of his second wife, Elizabeth Pole. Thus, these two famous Victorian scientists are not quite cousins germane. The following is hardly germane to the story, but it concerns sex, and sex we will all agree is more interesting than statistics, so we shall not skip it. When Mary Howard died, some 11 years were to pass before Erasmus married Elizabeth Pole. The intervening years were partly taken up by his fathering illegitimate children by another woman and partly in waiting for Mr. Pole, who was thirty years Elizabeth's senior, to depart this life and clear the stage for a successor, Erasmus, who had been writing passionate poetry to Elizabeth in the meantime.

Galton was to share his famous cousin's interest in heredity. However, whereas Charles was to make a name by considering precisely that aspect of genetic inheritance that was *not* preserved in the offspring, evolutionary innovation, and the mechanism of natural selection by which such innovation might be encouraged, Galton was to concentrate on that which was preserved. Indeed, it was to become something of an obsession to him.

But it was only one of his fixations. Galton was also obsessed with statistics and, although a very poor mathematician, had a combination of determination, instinct, flair and indefatigable enthusiasm for measuring anything and everything that caused him to make discoveries that others more able in analysis overlooked. We have already encountered his investigations into the inheritance of stature. His investigations of the height of parents and children, in leading to the discovery of regression to the mean, were of a profound importance he could not possibly have suspected when setting out to obtain his data. Another of his projects was to produce a feminine beauty map of Britain. He wandered the streets of Britain with a cross in his pocket and a pricker (no sniggering at the back please) with which he made a mark at the top of the cross whenever he passed a beauty, the longer bottom arm being reserved for ugly women and the lateral arms for those of indifferent pulchritude. By this means he discovered that for Britain London provided the zenith of beauty and Aberdeen the nadir; one cannot but speculate as to whether the tendency of some Scots to wear a kilt did not confuse his statistics.

Galton was independently wealthy. His grandfather Samuel Galton had made a fortune from gun manufacture, which activity he improbably combined with being a devout Quaker. However, whatever else Francis ultimately inherited from his grandfather, religion was not of the party. Francis was a convinced atheist at a time when it was not fashionable and given his obsessions it is hardly surprising that he brought statistics to bear on his non beliefs. We now consider an investigation that he made of the efficacy of prayer.

Praying for reign

In a paper that Francis eventually published, with some difficulty, in the *Fortnightly Review*,[11] he considered various forms of statistical evidence for the efficacy of prayer. He writes, true statistician that he is, 'There are two lines of research, by either of which we may pursue this inquiry. The one that promises the most trustworthy results is to examine large classes of cases, and to be guided by broad averages; the other, which I will not employ in these pages, is to deal with isolated instances.'[12] He then adds, 'An inquiry . . . may be made into the longevity of persons whose lives are prayed for; . . . . The public prayer for the sovereign of every state, Protestant and Catholic'.

He then pulls a trick that is a continuing favourite of statisticians, namely to analyse somebody else's data. Many supposedly applied statisticians have no interest whatsoever in collecting data and live a parasitical existence, appropriating for their uses sets that have already been collected by others. For example, in the field of multiple regression, there are dozens of papers providing yet another analysis of Brownlee's famous 'stack-loss' data,[13] which describe the operation of a chemical plant. (A review article by Dodge[14] written in 1997 identifies at least 90.) Anderson's Iris data were used by R. A. Fisher to illustrate discriminant functions[15] and have been used by just about everybody else working in 'multivariate analysis' since for the same purpose. The Canadian Lynx data, originally analysed by Moran,[16] have become a favourite in the subject known as time-series. However, as we have already explained, Galton was no slouch in collecting data. Here, however, he had a gift that was too good to pass up. Data had been collected by Dr. William A. Guy and published in the *Journal of the Statistical Society of London*.[17] Guy (1810–1885), who was professor of forensic medicine at King's College,[18] was a founding fellow of what later became the Royal Statistical Society, and an indefatigable collector of data concerning mortality and other epidemiological matters. The Society's prestigious 'Guy medals' are named after him. An extract of Galton's summary of Guy's data, together with his heading for it, is given in Table 6.1.[19] Galton writes, 'The sovereigns are literally the shortest lived of all who have the advantage of affluence. The prayer has therefore no

Table 6.1. *Mean age attained by males of various classes who had survived their 30th year, from 1758 to 1843. Deaths by accident are excluded.*

	In number	Average
Members of Royal houses	97	64.04
English aristocracy	1179	67.31
Gentry	1632	70.22

efficacy, unless the very questionable hypothesis be raised, that the conditions of royal life may naturally be yet more fatal, and that their influence is partly, though incompletely, neutralised by the effects of public prayers'.

Galton is using here a standard epidemiologist's device. A group is chosen who differ as regards the exposure in question but who are otherwise as similar as possible. The exposure here is, 'being prayed for'. This method is usually regarded as being second best to the randomised clinical trial. In the RCT we 'walk the talk'. Patients or subjects are first assembled together. Whether or not the patients are homogenous as a group, we are agreed on one thing. Any one of them can be given either of the two treatments and we then proceed to demonstrate that this is so by deciding completely at random who will receive what.

Where this cannot be done, there is always the possibility of hidden bias. The problem of 'confounding factors' or 'confounders' is, in fact, regarded as being the central difficulty of epidemiology. It is interesting to see that Galton is aware of this. He comments on the possible objection to his conclusion, that the results are biased by the hidden confounding effect of a more dangerous lifestyle that prayers partly counteract. Of course his discussion does not really meet this objection and moreover he is being slightly disingenuous, since Guy himself, based on his observations that agricultural workers were particularly long-lived, had proposed the theory that a sedentary life of luxury was unhealthy.

Blind faith

It might be supposed that it would be impossible to conduct a clinical trial of the efficacy of prayer. However, Dick Joyce, who was a colleague of mine for some years when I worked for CIBA-Geigy in Basle, once collaborated in designing a prospective blind trial of prayer.[20] Patients were matched in pairs and one member of each pair was assigned to be prayed for, the other acting as a control. Neither the patient nor the patient's physician knew which group the patient was assigned to. The 'treatment' was to receive a total of 15 hours prayer over a 6-month period. The trial was run as a sequential trial, results being updated as each pair reached the end of the treatment period.

The study was stopped after 19 pairs had been treated, at which point the results were just short of a boundary, which, had it been crossed, would have allowed one to declare a 'significant' benefit of prayer.

The results are thus perfectly consistent with all viewpoints and this, perhaps more than anything, can be taken as evidence of Divine Providence.

Clearly, where such manipulation of treatment is not possible, we have difficulty in convincing all critics of a causal relationship (or sometimes a lack of it), whatever the exposure being investigated. This has been the situation with smoking and lung cancer. For obvious practical and ethical reasons, it has been impossible to randomise schoolchildren either to smoke or not to smoke and follow them over their lifetimes. Consequently, it has been argued that the very strong association that has consistently been found between smoking and lung cancer is not convincing evidence that the former is a cause of the latter. Before we have a look at some of the alternative explanations, we divert to consider a key study that helped establish the association.

Smoke without fire?[21]

A custom loathsome to the eye, hateful to the nose, harmful to the brain, dangerous to the lungs, and in the black, stinking fume thereof, nearest resembling the horrible Stygian smoke of the pit that is bottomless.

James I & VI, *A Counterblaste to Tobacco*

No wonder King James disliked Sir Walter Raleigh. Perhaps we need look no further for the reason he had him beheaded.[22] However, excellent though the many reasons are of 'the wisest fool in Christendom', for the terrible effects of tobacco, they are not statistical and this, at least as far as this book is concerned, is a sad deficiency.

Two landmark papers of the effects of smoking and lung cancer are generally taken to be the study by Austin Bradford Hill and Richard Doll,[23] published in the *British Medical Journal* of 1950 and that of Wynder and Graham, published in the *Journal of the American Medical Association* in the same year.[24] In fact, an earlier important study had been carried out in Nazi Germany by Schairer and Schniger.[25] This was overlooked for many years for understandable political and sociological reasons but has recently been rediscovered by George Davey Smith and Mathias Eggar. In fact, warnings about the effects of smoking on health pre-date not only the Hill and Doll study but also that by Schairer by decades. The case against smoking has never been entirely forgotten since the time of King James. We concentrate here, however, on the paper by Doll and Hill.

This was a case–control study. The key feature of a case–control study is that sampling of data is by outcome. That is to say we choose to examine cases and controls and compare them in terms of exposure. In their study Doll and Hill sampled cases of lung cancer from four hospitals in the United Kingdom and compared them to a similar number of controls, who were patients admitted for other reasons. The common alternative approach, a cohort study, would identify smokers and non-smokers and count how many of each got lung cancer and how many did not. Conceptually, cohort studies follow subjects over time and are thus often referred to as *prospective* whereas case–control studies are referred to as *retrospective*, since observation of exposure takes place after determination of disease status.

At odds with life

The data that Doll and Hill assembled were as follows.

	Cases	Controls	Total
Smoker	1350	1296	2646
Non-smoker	7	61	68
Total	1357	1357	2714

The table suggests a rather different pattern as regards smoking status for cases and controls. This is not so much evident from inspecting the numbers of smokers as by looking at the number of non-smokers, where the figure of 7 is strikingly different from that of 61.

A problem with case–control data is that we have no idea as to how many smokers one has to follow to get one case. However, by looking at the problem in terms of odds rather than probabilities this difficulty is overcome. Remember that odds are a ratio of probabilities. Now suppose that we consider the population who contributed the lung-cancer cases. That is we consider conceptually the population of persons who would be admitted to the four hospitals studied by Doll and Hill if they were suffering from lung cancer during the time that the cases were collected. Suppose that this population is of size P_1. Treating proportions as probabilities, the probability of a member of this population being a smoker and having lung cancer is $1350/P_1$. On the other hand, the probability of being a non-smoker and having lung cancer is $7/P_1$. If the ratio of one to the other is calculated, the unknown divisor P_1 cancels out and in this instance we are left with odds of $1350/7 = 193$. Similarly by considering the conceptual population of controls or non-cases, P_2, we can estimate the odds of being a smoker in a way that eliminates the unknown P_2 as $1296/61 = 21$. The ratio of one set of odds to the other is the odds-ratio and in this case this equals $193/21 = 9$. So that the odds of being a smoker amongst cases is nine times as high as the odds amongst controls.

Now look at this in a slightly different way. Suppose that I wish to calculate the odds of a smoker getting lung cancer, $Odds_S$, compared to some other illness. This is then (conceptually) given by the ratio of two proportions involving the two unknown populations as follows,

$$Odds_S = \frac{(1350/P_1)}{(1296/P_2)} = \left(\frac{1350}{1296}\right)\left(\frac{P_2}{P_1}\right).$$

Unfortunately the unknown population values do not disappear from this. However, I can calculate a similar quantity, $Odds_N$, for non-smokers as

$$Odds_N = \frac{(7/P_1)}{(61/P_2)} = \left(\frac{7}{61}\right)\left(\frac{P_2}{P_1}\right).$$

Now if I calculate the ratio of the one set of odds to the other, the unknown ratio of populations P_2/P_1 cancels out to leave me with

$$OR = \left(\frac{1350}{1296}\right)\left(\frac{61}{7}\right) = 9$$

as before. Thus the odds ratio (OR) can also be interpreted as the ratio of the odds of a smoker getting lung cancer to the odds of a non-smoker getting lung cancer.

Risky business

The odds scale, especially when log-transformed, is a favourite amongst statisticians, whether or not its use is forced by the exigencies of the sampling scheme, as with case–control studies. This is because of its useful statistical properties. However, its interpretation may be more difficult. In fact, provided that the disease is rare, the odds ratio corresponds roughly to a ratio of probabilities. Even amongst smokers lung cancer is a rare disease so that the odds ratio here is also approximately the relative risk. We can thus say that the Doll and Hill data suggest that a smoker is nine times as likely to get lung cancer as a non-smoker.

There are of course several reasons for being cautious when faced with such data. For example, a pretty strong assumption has to be made about the way that cases and controls arise. Suppose that differences in social class, geographic distribution or policy led smokers with lung cancer to be treated in different hospitals to non-smokers with lung cancer, whereas for the diseases represented by the controls no such differentiation applies. Doll and Hill might have picked the wrong hospitals. Or suppose lung cancer to be a disease with a very uncertain diagnosis but that the knowledge that the putative sufferer is a smoker is much more likely to produce a diagnosis of lung cancer. One very plausible source of bias will, if anything, lead to an underestimate of risk. This is the possibility, since suggested by many further studies, that smoking also predisposes to other diseases apart from cancer. If this is true, patients suffering from other diseases are a far from ideal control group. The business of finding suitable controls remains a central difficulty of case–control studies.

The critics were not slow in lining up to take pot-shots at Doll and Hill. In due course, they were to face some very big guns indeed. Amongst the shells lobbed at them were several from R. A. Fisher.

Fisher's angle

Two of Fisher's arguments posited alternative explanations for the association. First, he suggested that lung cancer could be a disease that developed early in adolescence and developed extremely slowly. This made it possible that lung cancer was the cause of smoking. The symptoms of lung cancer might encourage persons to take up smoking as a source of relief. A second argument proposed that there could be some common factor predisposing to both smoking and lung cancer. He suggested, for example, that there could be a gene for wanting to smoke that was associated with the gene for lung cancer.[26]

Of course there may also be a gene for making statements of this sort associated with accepting money from tobacco companies. Fisher certainly accepted such money. However, I am convinced that this was not his motive in attacking Doll and Hill. Fisher had a cussed nature and a taste for disputation. I believe he was attracted by the challenge of proving Bradford Hill wrong.

He dismissed the observation that lung cancer had been rising rapidly in a period that had seen a rapid increase in smoking, by pointing out that the rapid increase in smoking amongst women was not accompanied by a similar increase. In a subsequent paper Fisher made much of the fact that in the Doll and Hill study the expected association between inhaling and lung cancer did not appear (dividing smokers up between those who inhaled and those who did not). He also pointed out the limitations of studies that were not randomised (whilst stressing that this was an inherent limitation of the field, requiring circumspection in drawing conclusions, and not an adverse comment on researchers in it).

This latter criticism, however valid and politely put, was pure hypocrisy. Fisher himself was rarely involved in purely medical matters. Most of his important work was theoretical and that which was not related primarily to agriculture or genetics. However, a rare foray of his into medicine was described in a joint paper with W. R. B. Atkins, 'the therapeutic use of vitamin C',[27] as follows. 'Observations made upon two sections of R. A. M. C. men dosed with vitamin C gave differences far beyond those that could be attributed to chance. It was ascertained that men of one section were dosed before breakfast, those of the other after it. The latter became saturated and excreted vitamin sooner than the former.'

In fact, not only was this study not randomised, all the men given vitamin C before breakfast being in one section and those given it after in another, this was not even a study designed to answer the question Atkins and Fisher were now asking. The original study had the purpose of examining the vitamin C reserves of troops. It was purely by chance and not by design that vitamin C was given according to two different regimes. 'The same hospital was visited four months later and further inquiries elicited that the section A men of the R. A. M. C. had paraded at 07.30 hrs., before breakfast, having been busy attending to patients. Section B men, finding they were not required immediately, had their food and received the dose of vitamin C afterwards. The routine was followed on subsequent days. It appears therefore that vitamin C is much better utilized after other foods which is in keeping with the custom of having dessert after meals.'

In criticising Hill and Doll, Fisher was throwing stones from his glasshouse.

Physician heal thyself

Interestingly, Fisher's criticisms are not so much of the case–control methodology itself, in the sense of stressing the biases of the case–control approach compared to the prospective cohort approach time. His criticisms are of the sort that apply to all observational studies, whether cohort or case–control, compared to randomised interventions. This was, perhaps, because he was covering his back for further results that were to arrive. By the time Fisher wrote his criticisms a cohort study of British

doctors, initiated by Doll and Hill, was well under way and prelimi-
nary reports had been obtained. This was a brilliant stroke of Hill's, who
recognised that doctors might make a particularly good group to study.
In October 1951 a postal questionnaire was sent to all men and women
recorded on the British medical register, inquiring about their smoking
habits. Usable replies were received from 34 439 men and 6194 women.
Follow-up studies have been carried out at various intervals, although
these have concentrated on the men, due to the initial rarity of female
smokers.

This long-running cohort study has not only confirmed the findings of
the original case–control study but also made it clear that this biased the
estimate of the risk of lung–cancer downwards, as discussed above, due to
the adverse effect of smoking on health in other areas and hence its effect
on the hospital controls in the original study.[28] Of course, this would not
disprove Fisher's genetic hypothesis. Attempts have been made to answer
this in other ways. A Finnish study obtained, with what must have been
great difficulty, data on 22 monozygotic (that is to say identical) twins that
were discordant for smoking status[29] (that is to say, where one smoked and
the other did not). In 17 out of the 22 pairs the smoker died first. Excluding the remote possibility of simultaneous death, the probability of the
smoker dying first under the null hypothesis of no effect of smoking is 0.5.
The probability of 17 or more such cases is found from the binomial distribution with $n = 22$ and $p = 0.5$ to be 0.0085, which if we double it gives
us a P-value of 0.017. In other words only about 2 in 100 collections of 22
such pairs of twins would be expected to show a discrepancy in favour or
against non-smokers as great as this. This is highly suggestive but not conclusive. In fact, only two of the deaths were of lung cancer (both to smokers), reflecting, no doubt, its rarity as a disease. There was a 9 (smokers)
to 0 (non-smokers) split in terms of death from heart disease and a 6 to 5
split from other causes. Research since the early fifties comparing smokers with non-smokers has shown that although the odds ratio for getting
lung cancer is much higher than that for heart disease, the excess risk is
much greater for heart disease because the latter is much more common.

Since Fisher died, and perhaps because many have been more impressed by Doll and Hill's arguments than by his, a natural experiment
has been underway. In many developed countries there has been a falling
off in the proportion of male smokers and at long last a reduction in
cancer death rates for males has appeared. However, smoking rates in
women have been rising to meet the falling rates in men and the failure

of lung cancer to increase in women, to which Fisher drew attention, is a failure no more, although the phenomenon does represent a failure of public health.

Ashes to ashes

Fisher was a genius, a brilliant and profound thinker, and an important innovator, not just in statistics but also in genetics and evolutionary biology. Bradford Hill was a truly great epidemiologist and medical statistician but neither as a scientist nor as a mathematician was he in Fisher's class. However, on the matter of smoking, in the years that have elapsed since their dispute, Bradford Hill's arguments look better and better and Fisher's more and more foolish. As the American biostatistician Jerome Cornfield pointed out,[30] to explain away the hypothesis that smoking caused lung cancer you had to make appeal to hidden factors whose action was even stronger than the putative effect of smoking (since they were unlikely to split 100% smokers, 0% non-smokers). The more pieces of the puzzle appeared, the less plausible the alternative explanations appeared. In contributing to the debate, Fisher had chosen to be clever rather than wise and this choice was neither.

7

Time's tables

I read the tables drawn wi' care
For an Insurance Company,
Her chance o' life was stated there,
Wi' perfect perspicuity.

George Outram, The Annuity

Unhappy returns

The man in George Outram's poem sells an old lady an annuity, relying on an insurance company's life-table to set the price. Unfortunately she beats the mean and years later he is left bemoaning the fact that he still has to pay her her annuity, the premium being long gone.

But tables here or tables there,
She's lived ten years beyond her share,
An's like to live a dozen mair,
To ca' for her annuity.

In setting premiums for life insurance, annuities and so forth, one has to be careful about two matters. The first is that the premiums should be set at a level that will not leave the insurer out of pocket in the long run. The second is that the fund is secure against a run of possible bad luck. This latter issue is known as the problem of gambler's ruin and is a very old one in statistics, having formed one of the subjects of Pascal's famous exchange of letters with Fermat.[1] It was also treated by Christiaan Huygens in the book John Arbuthnot translated into English, *De Ratiociniis in Ludo Aleae* (1657).[2] Given a very large number of persons insured, provided that life expectancies and other quantities related to them have been calculated correctly, the contingency required in percentage terms to cover a run against the fund is small. This fact is the justification for insurance. The members of an insurance fund protect each other by virtue of their number. Outram's insurer was unlucky but he only appears to have had one client and so the result is not so remarkable.

But how do we decide on expectation of life? This is, indeed, a matter that has occupied a number of mathematicians, scientists, and actuaries over the centuries. In this chapter we consider some early attempts at constructing life-tables as well as the way in which this particular topic has been most remarkably extended and modified by statisticians in the last thirty or forty years.

Time gentlemen, please

The basic idea behind a modern life-table is to take some imaginary cohort of individuals and follow their progress to the grave. Usually a convenient number such as 1000 or 100 000 is used and this is referred to as the radix of the table. This is the root at which time and mortality will gnaw. The rate of attrition is determined by reference to data from some convenient or relevant population. From these data death rates can be calculated and from death rates probabilities of dying (the two are not quite the same as will be explained in due course). These probabilities are then applied year by year (and usually separately for each sex) to the current survivors to determine who will see their next birthday and who will have just seen their last.

The mortality experience thus constructed is usually theoretical and not of direct relevance to any actual generation of persons, since the data are almost always constructed from a given calendar period. Thus, for example, if we construct a life-table for the USA using deaths and population figures for the year 2000, the death rates for 90 year olds are calculated from those who were born before the First World War, whereas those from 30 years old are from a generation who weren't in a position to remember where they were when John F. Kennedy was shot.

In using such a life-table to calculate the expectation of life for a 30-year-old male, say, one is thus using death rates that will have less and less relevance the longer time goes on. To see the implications of this, imagine determining for an individual who has reached the age of 60 what his probability is of surviving to 65. One would hardly use probabilities based on data that were 30–40 years out of date, yet if his life was insured at age 30 up to age 65, these very same rates are amongst those that *will* have been used in writing *that* policy.

This fact has important consequences for the insurance business. The last century showed a dramatic increase in life-expectancy. This means that life insurance policies were generally a better bet for the insurer than annuities, since in the former case the returns live on with your client, whereas in the latter case your obligations die with him.

Deceased, Tunbridge Wells[3]*

Tunbridge Wells, as we saw in Chapter 2, was where Thomas Bayes was a minister when he wrote his famous treatise. This has nothing to do with its appearance here. Queen Anne – who, through her indefatigable production of short-lived progeny, must have done more than any other monarch to depress the expectation of life for royalty – complained about the dangerous conditions underfoot in Tunbridge Wells on a Royal visit to what was to become the Pantiles.[4] John Arbuthnot was her physician. None of this is of relevance either. What is relevant, however, is that it just so happens that my first job was working for the Tunbridge Wells Health District (1975–1978) and during my time there I constructed a life-table for the District, which I now propose to discuss.

As is the modern practice, I produced a separate table for males and females. I hope that the good ladies of Tunbridge Wells will forgive me, but for reasons of brevity I shall present the results for gentlemen only. These are given in Table 7.1.

The values are at five-year intervals and each row is deemed to apply to an individual male who has the exact age given by the first column. The second column gives the probability that a given male will fail to see five further birthdays. The radix of the table is the first entry in the third column and is 100 000, so we can imagine that we follow 100 000 males from birth. Subsequent entries give the numbers of the original 'cohort' of 100 000 who survive to the given age. By multiplying this number by the corresponding value of qx we can calculate how many we expect to die before the next row of the table is reached and this gives us the number of deaths, dx. Thus, for example, 77 115 survive to age 65, their probability of dying before age 70 is 0.1571 so that $0.1571 \times 77\,115 = 12\,115$ are expected to die in the five years between exact ages 65 and 70. Obviously, by subtracting this number from the current entry in the lx column we get the next entry. Thus, $77\,115 - 12\,115 = 65\,000$. In this way all the values in columns three and four can be constructed starting with the first entry of column three (100 000) and using the appropriate values of qx in column two.

Table 7.1. *Life expectancy for males, Tunbridge Wells Health District, 1971.*

Age X	qx	lx	dx	Lx	Tx	Ex
0	0.0160	100 000	1600	496 000	7 204 449	72.0
5	0.0012	98 400	118	491 705	6 708 449	68.2
10	0.0006	98 282	59	491 262	6 216 744	63.3
15	0.0029	98 223	285	490 403	5 725 482	58.3
20	0.0055	97 938	539	488 344	5 235 079	53.5
25	0.0043	97 399	419	485 950	4 746 735	48.7
30	0.0037	96 981	359	484 006	4 260 785	43.9
35	0.0052	96 622	502	481 853	3 776 779	39.1
40	0.0044	96 119	423	479 540	3 294 926	34.3
45	0.0186	95 696	1 780	474 032	2 815 386	29.4
50	0.0327	93 916	3 071	461 905	2 341 354	24.9
55	0.0611	90 845	5 551	440 350	1 879 449	20.7
60	0.0959	85 295	8 180	406 024	1 439 099	16.9
65	0.1571	77 115	12 115	355 288	1 033 075	13.4
70	0.2420	65 000	15 730	285 676	677 786	10.4
75	0.3773	49 270	18 590	199 877	392 110	8.0
80	0.4984	30 681	15 291	115 175	192 234	6.3
85	0.6075	15 389	9 349	53 574	77 059	5.0
90	0.7224	6 040	4 364	19 293	23 485	3.9
95	1	1 677	1 677	4 192	4 192	2.5

The fifth column, headed Lx, is the total number years of life lived in the given five-year interval, assuming an even distribution of deaths in the interval, which assumption is *fairly* appropriate for the early years of life, with the exception of the first, but becomes progressively less so as age increases. (Refinements are possible but are not illustrated here.) Thus we argue as follows. There were 77 115 alive aged 65 and 65 000 aged 70. On average there were (77 115 + 65 000)/2 = 71 057.5 persons and so the years of life lived were 5 × 71057.5 = 355 288 (rounding up).

The sixth column, Tx, represents the total years of life lived beyond a given age by the cohort and so is calculated by summing the Lx values from the bottom of the table. Finally the expectation of further life is calculated at any age by dividing the expected total years of further life for the cohort at age *x*, Tx, by the number still alive to live them, lx. So for example we have that the expectation at 65 is 1 033 075/77 115 = 13.4.

Pretty deadly stuff*

Of course, all of this follows pretty trivially from the values of qx, even if their calculation in 1976, with the help of a desktop-calculator with a roll of paper to print out results, took a great deal more effort than I needed to repeat the exercise some 25 years later with the help of a spreadsheet. However, the real labour was in finding values of qx and this is the problem that all constructors of life-tables face.

First, the Tunbridge Wells Health District was a rather small unit of population consisting of some 196 000 persons, a little over 92 000 of whom were males. The average five-year age group thus had about 5000 males: rather more than this for some of the earlier age groups and rather less than this for the latter. However, the earlier age groups have low mortality so that the table is based on very few deaths at the lower end of the scale and subject to considerable random variation. To minimise this I combined deaths for 1970, 1971 and 1972.

For the calculation of national death rates, a mid-year population is estimated for a given year by the Office for National Statistics. I do not know whether this population is now estimated locally by age and sex (I suspect not) but such estimates were not available to me in 1976. This is why the year 1971, a census year, was chosen. The deaths over the three-year period had to be referred to a population that was actually counted on the night of 25/26 April 1971, which is not quite the middle of the three-year period and a weighting of the three years was introduced to reflect this. By referring the weighted annual average to the population alive, it was then possible to calculate death rates.

The death rate, however, is not quite the same as the probability of dying, even allowing for the fact that relative frequencies are not quite the same as probabilities. The death rate is the ratio of those who die during a year to the mid-year population. There are then two issues. The first is that the cohort of persons who contribute to the deaths is not exactly the same as the cohort who contribute to the population: the numerator is not perfectly coeval with the denominator. Consider the case of all males who died aged 63 in 1971. Their exact ages at death range from 63 years to nearly 64 years. The first born among them could have died just short of his 64th birthday on January 1, 1971. Such an individual was born on 2 January 1907. However, the last born amongst them could have died on his 63rd birthday on December 31, 1971. He was born on December 31, 1908. Thus we are talking of individuals who were born in a two-year period. However, suppose we were to refer them to the mid-year population (as we might be able to do when calculating a life-table at national level). These are all males aged 63 on 30 June, 1971. Clearly, they were born any time between 1 July, 1907 and 30 June, 1908. Thus we have a slightly different cohort. Provided the population is reasonably stable, however, in the sense that the number of 63 year olds is not changing much from one year to the next, this does not matter.

The second reason, however, is more important. Any individual who dies aged 63 before the mid-year date contributes to the numerator (the deaths) but not the denominator (the population). Suppose we start with 100 individuals and that 10 die in the first half of the year and 10 in the second half, so that the mid-year population is 90. The death rate per 1000 is $1000 \times {}^{20}/_{90} = 222$. On the other hand, the life-table probability of dying is the ratio of the deaths in the period to those alive at the beginning of the period and would thus be $20/100 = 0.2$, or, 200 if multiplied by 1000. Thus we see that death rates cannot be used directly for life-tables. Of course, given an assumption of the way that deaths are distributed throughout the age group in question, it is possible to estimate one from the other and there are actuarial tables to do this.

This computational matter is pretty deadly stuff; it is time that we had some light relief, and where better to find light than by looking at the sky?

Edmond Halley (1656–1742)

Halley was the son of a wealthy soap-boiler.[5] He was already a keen amateur astronomer as a schoolboy and when he went up to Oxford in 1673 he brought with him a collection of astronomical instruments. He left Oxford without a degree and in November 1676, aged 20, embarked for St. Helena where he stayed for nearly two years, producing an accurate catalogue of the southern sky. On his return he was awarded a degree at Oxford and made a Fellow of the Royal Society. Amongst his contemporaries his St. Helena trip made his reputation as an astronomer but this was sealed for posterity with a prediction that was posthumously made good. The great comet of 1682 inspired him to compute the orbits of 24 comets. The comets of 1456, 1531, 1607 and 1682 had very similar orbits. Halley concluded they were the same and predicted a return in 1758. A comet obligingly reappeared in 1758, by which time its herald was 16 years dead, and it now bears Halley's name.

Halley made important contributions to astronomy and physics in his own right but is also important for the help he gave Newton in the production of the *Principia*.[6] 'He paid all the expenses, he corrected the proofs, he laid aside all his own work in order to press forward to the utmost to the printing.'[7]

It will not be obvious to the reader, however, as to why we have taken time off from the actuarial to discuss the astronomical. Patience! All will be revealed shortly. However, for the moment, we shall recede on an elliptical peregrination, returning, comet-like, to our appointment with Halley in due course.

Life, but not as we know it[8]

I have taken the pains, and been at the charge, of setting out those Tables, whereby all men may both correct my Positions, and raise others of their own: For herein I have, like a silly Scholeboy, coming to say my Lesson to the World (that Peevish, and Tetchie Master) brought a bundle of Rods wherewith to be whipt, for every mistake I have committed.

John Graunt[9]

Those who ordered the affairs of Breslau in Silesia at the end of the sixteenth century were wise men, fully cognisant of the value of statistics, for they commanded that a register be kept of births by sex and of deaths by sex and age. When searching for evidence to combat superstitions, the scientist and pastor Caspar Neumann (1648–1715) used these data to show that the phases of the Moon had no influence on health and also that the 'grand climacticum' years of 49 and 63 were not particularly dangerous. He sent his results to Leibniz who in turn communicated them to the Royal Society in 1689.

The Society had itself been interested in the matter, due to the labours of one of its fellows. But to understand these labours we need to know something of the history of English vital statistics. In 1538, Thomas Cromwell introduced a system of parish registers of weddings, christenings and burials for members of the Church of England.[10] He did not have to wait long to contribute personally to the latter, since he was executed by Henry VIII two years later. Perhaps he ought to have included divorces in the vital statistics. From 1604 the Company of Parish Clerks published weekly bills of mortality and annual summaries for London. From 1625 these were printed. Although age at death was not recorded untill 1728, from 1629 onwards numbers of christenings and burials were recorded separately for males and females and this explains why the series that John Arbuthnot used for his significance test started in that year. However, as far as we are aware, no serious attempt was made to analyse these data before 1662, when John Graunt (1620–1674), the son of a draper, published a remarkable book, *Natural and Political Observations Made upon the Bills of*

Mortality. The book eventually ran to five editions and Graunt managed the rare trick of making a best-seller out of statistics. (I cannot contemplate Graunt's success without envy!). The book, together with a helpful recommendation from Charles II, secured his election to the newly founded Royal Society.

Graunt's statistical investigations are extremely wide-ranging. He noted, for example, the sex ratio at birth and its stability that was to form the basis of Arbuthnot's probabilistic treatment. He also established that burials exceeded christenings in London, and that this excess had increased, due to changing religious attitudes towards the value of christening. However, we are interested in him here because, with great difficulty, he constructed a crude life-table.

The reason for his difficulty was that the ages at death were not recorded. However as Graunt explains, 'The *Searchers* hereupon (who are antient Matrons, sworn to their office) repair to the place, where the dead Corps lies, and by view of the same, and by other enquiries, they examine by what *Disease,* or *Casualty* the Corps died.' Graunt used these causes of death to estimate how many persons died in given age ranges. (For example, he could identify certain causes as diseases of infancy.) From this he was able to construct a crude life-table.

Graunt's book created considerable interest but it also raised the question as to whether one might do better. To do this required better data, in particular data on ages at death. These were now available thanks to the foresight of the wise men of Breslau and the interests of Caspar Neumann. The assistant secretary of the Royal Society and the editor of its journal, *Philosophical Transactions*, took up the task of seeing what might be done. His name was Edmond Halley.

From orbits to obits

This City of *Breslaw* is the Capital City of the Province of *Silesia*; or, as the *Germans* call it, *Schlesia*, and is situated on the Western Bank of the River *Oder*, anciently called *Viadrus*; near the Confines of *Germany* and *Poland*, and very near the Latitude of *London*.

Edmond Halley[11]

Haley makes no distinction of sex but uses average deaths by age for the data Neumann had collected. These are for the five years 1687–1691. In this period, 'there were born 6193 Persons, and buried 5869'. He reduces these to annual averages of 1238 and 1174. If he could assume that the population

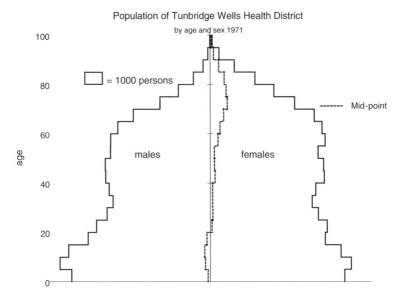

Figure 7.1 Population pyramid for the Tunbridge Wells Health District 1971 by age and sex.

was stable, there would be no difficulty in constructing his life-table. The average age of those who died would be the expectation of life at birth.[12] However where the population is not stable such an approach is biased. Suppose for example that the birth rate is higher than the death rate and the population is growing year by year. The deaths of the young are a fraction of a larger population than are the deaths of the old. Young deaths will thus be over-represented and we will underestimate the expectation of life.

The 'population pyramid' in Figure 7.1, which is for the Tunbridge Wells Health district 1971, illustrates the sort of thing that happens in real populations. (I never published this work and intend to get value out of it now!) Note that there are actually more males and females alive between ages 40 and 50 than between ages 30 and 40. This is a situation which cannot arrive in a life-table population where each successive age group must contain fewer individuals. (The pyramid also illustrates Arbuthnot's divine providence admirably. The closer the dashed line, which represents the mid-point, is to the solid vertical one, the more evenly the sexes are balanced. Note how wonderfully an excess of males is translated into just the right number when women reach marriageable age.)

However, Halley does not have population figures and thus, although in a much better position than Graunt who did not even have age at death but had to infer this, cannot proceed as I was able to do with the population of Tunbridge Wells. He starts by assuming that he somehow has to account for what will happen to the 1238 births using the deaths from the 1174. The difference between these two figures is 64. He states that from the table available to him it seems that 348 die in the first year of life. This leaves him with 890. He also states that in the next five years 198 will die and distributes their number evenly amongst the period. This would leave him with 692 survivors at age 6. Now, however, he produces a distribution of deaths by age for the remaining years based on the actual deaths observed and this only adds up to 628, the difference to 692 being the 64 already noted.

Next by a less than transparent procedure he somehow reconciles these figures and produces his life-table. Unlike the modern form this does not use the imaginary device of a cohort, the radix, starting life together on the same date, but gives the actual number alive in Breslau in the first year. This is the equivalent of the Lx figure in a modern life-table rather than the lx figure. (See the example of Tunbridge Wells, where however, the age groups are of five years width rather than one as used by Halley.) The figure Halley gives is 1000. This can be interpreted in two ways. Either as a convenient number to start with, or as pretty much the true figure for Breslau given the fact that according to Halley's estimate out of 1238 born only '890 do arrive at a full Years Age'. The average of 1238 and 890 is 1064 but bearing in mind that more infants will die in the first weeks than towards the end of the year, the number of years of life lived will be lower than this and might plausibly be very close to 1000.

We shall not discuss Halley's life-table further but give a graphical representation in Figure 7.2. below. Instead we shall take a leap of some three centuries. However, a leap of this length is not without its hazards and indeed the so-called *hazard rate* is what will have to discuss. We need to make ourselves better acquainted with it first.

Time's winged chariot

A key epidemiological concept in understanding risk is 'person-time at risk', sometimes loosely referred to as exposure. (This was implicit, for example, in the discussion of Viagra in Chapter 6.) It is often approximately true, under conditions we shall consider in due course, that the number of

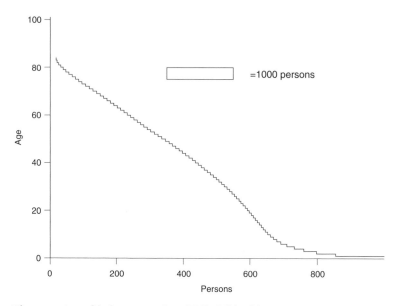

Figure 7.2 A graphical representation of Halley's life-table.

deaths we expect to see in a population is proportional to the person-time at risk. For example, in similar populations, we should expect to see approximately the same number of deaths if we studied 10 000 persons for a year or 120 000 for a month. In each case the person-years of exposure are 10 000.

Of course, if the observation time is increased considerably, this is not true. In most populations the death rate increases with increasing age. Hence if we follow a group of 10 000 individuals for 30 years we shall expect to see more deaths than if we follow an initially comparable group of 300 000 individuals for one year. As we have already seen, such a group is referred to by epidemiologists as a *cohort*, a collective noun that (singular) originally meant a tenth part of a Roman legion but now (*plural*) seems to be used increasingly in the newspapers to mean persons accompanying another, as in, 'Madonna appeared at the party surrounded by her cohorts'. Thus hacks have now added to their inability to understand the basics of the statistics of cohorts an inability to understand the word: at sea with both signifier and signified. What can it be a sign of?

The conditions to which we referred above, which make the expected number of deaths proportional to exposure, are that the so-called *hazard rate* should be both constant and small. The hazard rate is the probability of dying within a small interval given that one has survived so far. To make this obscure statement clear, we shall have no choice but to play a simple game of chance. Since death is our subject and we wish to relieve some Stygian gloom, tossing a coin, Charon's toll in this case, might be appropriate. It was such a coin that the musician Jeremiah Clarke, disappointed in love, tossed to decide whether to drown himself in a pond he was passing. It fell with its side imbedded in the mud, so he went home and blew his brains out. But edge-up coins are too fantastical for a work such as this, where all is probability, and 50:50 is too symmetrical, too even, too boring. Let us increase the odds of survival and consider a game of Russian roulette.

Revolver

I am the one in ten
A number on a list
I am the one in ten
Even though I don't exist
Nobody knows me
Even though I'm always there
A statistic, a reminder
Of a world that doesn't care

UB40, *One in Ten*[13]

Take a revolver with a chamber with space for six bullets, leave five spaces empty but put a bullet in the other, spin the chamber, place the gun to your head and pull the trigger. This brainless form of entertainment is a good way of hurrying along John Maynard Keynes's long run, which we discussed in the last chapter, but we shall use it not so much to illustrate the inevitability of death but the calculation of probabilities.

Suppose that you have a one in ten chance of propelling a live bullet through your head on the first shot. 'Wait a minute,' I hear the reader say, 'one in ten; don't you mean one in six?'. Not necessarily. That would be to use a vulgar argument of symmetry. Who said we were going to use classical probability? It is possible that the weight of the bullet is more likely to bring the chamber to rest at the bottom, whereas egress to the barrel is at the top. Of course, I have no empirical basis for my one in ten but I am in charge here and I like these odds better. One in ten it is.

Clearly the probability that the player will die on the first game is $1/10$. On the other hand if we wish to consider the probability that the player will die on the second game this is $(9/10) \times (1/10) = 0.09$ because we require him to survive the first game, which he will do with probability $9/10$ and then expire on the second, which he will do with probability $1/10$. Suppose, now, that we wish to calculate the probability that a player playing Russian Roulette will die on the third game? We may proceed as follows. In order to die on the third game he has to survive the first game and the second. The probability that he survives the first is $9/10$ and likewise for the second given that he lives to play it. Thus the probability of his surviving both games is $(9/10) \times (9/10)$. His probability of surviving both games and dying on the third is $(9/10) \times (9/10) \times (1/10) = 81/1000 = 0.081$.

The reader will now be hoping that this game will not carry on indefinitely and that our would-be suicide will soon achieve his desired end. There are only so many probability calculations of this sort that one can take before ennui sets is and one is tempted to seek dangerous distractions, possibly involving revolvers, who knows, as an alternative. However, algebra can come to our aid and it is not hard to find a general rule that will give us the probability that the individual will expire on a given number of attempts. Let us call that number n. In order to expire on the nth attempt the individual has to have survived $n - 1$ attempts, each of which he will do with probability $(9/10)$, the probability of surviving these being just $(9/10) \times (9/10) \ldots (9/10)$, where $n - 1$ such numbers are written, so that this probability is $(9/10)^n - 1$. We now have to multiply this by the probability of his expiring on the nth attempt having survived thus far, which is just $1/10$. Thus the overall probability of dying on attempt n is $(9/10)^{n-1} \times (1/10) = 9^{n-1}/10^n$.

What we have derived is the probability distribution of the number of attempts it takes for the individual to kill himself. If we wish to be more formal about this and write $p(n)$ for the probability that the individual dies at attempt n, then we may write

$$p(n) = \frac{9^{n-1}}{10^n}, \; n = 0, 1, \ldots$$

This handy formula now gives the probability of our dying on any occasion. To find out what our probability is of dying on the fifth shot we have to substitute $n = 5$ in the formula to obtain $p(5) = \frac{9^4}{10^5} = 0.66$. However, if we are interested in a rather different question, namely what is the probability of dying on or before the nth attempt, then this requires a different formula, one which represents the sum of the probabilities of dying on the first, the second and so forth up to the nth pull of the trigger. We will represent this probability by $F(n)$. The formula for this is simply derived by considering that the probability of our surviving up to and including the nth attempt, which we shall refer to as $S(n)$, is given by the product of our survival probabilities on each of the n occasions and so we have $S(n) = \left(\frac{9}{10}\right)^n$. However, we must either die on or before the nth attempt or survive up to and including the nth attempt. (We might refer to this as, 'the law of the excluded monster': Russian roulette players are either alive or dead but there are no undead.) Hence, $F(n) + S(n) = 1$ so that $F(n) = 1 - \left(\frac{9}{10}\right)^n$. For instance, our probability of dying on or before the fifth attempt is $F(5) = 1 - \left(\frac{9}{10}\right)^5 = 0.41$.

Now suppose we wish to calculate the probability of expiring on the nth attempt *given* that we have survived the first $n - 1$ attempts, which we shall refer to as $H(n)$. It is intuitively obvious (at least I hope that it is obvious) that this is simply $1/_{10}$. However, we can be tedious and formal about this and use Bayes theorem. This says that for any two events A and B the probability of A given B is the probability of A and B divided by the probability of B. Or, to put it algebraically, in a form we have already encountered, $P(A \mid B) = P(A \cap B)/P(B)$ where the symbol $\cap$ stands for 'and' and the symbol | stands for 'given'. Now, the probability of surviving the first $n - 1$ attempts and expiring on the nth attempt is simply the probability of expiring on the nth attempt, since this implies survival for the first $n - 1$ and this, we have already calculated, is $p(n) = \frac{9^{n-1}}{10^n}$. To calculate the probability of dying on the nth attempt given that we have survived $n - 1$, Bayes theorem tells us we need to divide this probability by $S(n - 1)$. However, since $S(n) = \left(\frac{9}{10}\right)^n$, $S(n - 1) = \left(\frac{9}{10}\right)^{n-1}$ so that we have

$$H(n) = p(n)/S(n-1) = \frac{\left(\frac{9^{n-1}}{10^n}\right)}{\left(\frac{9}{10}\right)^{n-1}} = \frac{1}{10}.$$

This long journey back to square one may seem pointless but it illustrates the general rule. By the instantaneous hazard rate we mean the probability of dying on a particular occasion (or in continuous time, at a given moment) given that one has survived so far and this can in general be calculated by dividing the probability of death on the occasion by the probability of surviving so far. The nearest life-table equivalent of this is qx. The equivalence is not perfect because the hazard rate is presumably changing continuously over time, yet we average it by using whole years, or in the case of my table five-year periods.

Note that there is no contradiction between a constant hazard and a declining probability of death. The probability of death on the fifth attempt is $p(5) = 0.066$. That of dying on the first is $p(1) = 0.1$. The former is lower than the latter; not because Russian roulette gets safer the more you play it. It does not. The appropriate measure of risk is the hazard rate and this is constant. The probability of dying on a given occasion has to cover the probability of having survived so far and this is lower for the 5th than for the first attempt. In the long run, our Rusian roulettist is almost surely dead. His probability of dying on a particular occasion given that he has survived so far is, however, constant. Of course hazard rates do not have to be constant and it is a general feature of life that, although they tend to reduce in the first few weeks of life, the general trend is for an increase as we get older.

The lessons for interpreting probability where time is concerned are: first, don't forget exposure and, second, be very careful to say exactly what sort of probability you are talking about if you intend to convey something meaningful.

Hazard a guess

If you go to the Web of Science (http://wos.mimas.ac.uk/) and do a citation search under Cox DR and the year 1972, you are offered a bewildering choice of articles. The list you get initially is not of papers that have cited the reference being sought but of papers produced by DR Cox in 1972. But can one man have written so many papers in one year? The list goes on for 10 pages with 20 papers per page. Once you are past the first few, however, you begin to realise that these are all suspiciously similar. A detail is changed here and there. Only once you get onto page 7 do you really understand what is going on. A paper by D. R. Cox[14] has been cited a staggering number of times: 15 759 citations when I looked it up on the 13 April 2002. In fact, it has been cited so many times that it has attracted a whole host of false citations. Many of these incorrect references have now acquired a life of their own and survive on as less successful but still viable mutations in this exploding population of references. I shall now attempt the difficult task of trying to explain exactly what it was that this paper achieved.

In order to do that we need to understand something about the different concerns of actuaries and medical statisticians. The former are more concerned to predict what will happen to those insured, since that affects contingent payments and hence premiums and profits. The latter are less concerned with what will happen but rather with what affects that which will happen. If patients are given beta-blockers do they live longer? Do smokers die younger and can we therefore conclude that if we can persuade smokers to give up their habit they will live longer?

The second point is that actuaries often deal with very large numbers.[15] This was not the case in the early days of the subject when, as we have seen, Halley had to construct his tables from a relatively small town in a far-off province. Now we have vital registration as part and parcel of the business of government and life-tables can be regularly produced and based on statistics collected from millions. In fact, as was pointed out in discussion of the Cox paper, fluctuations in the rate of interest are a greater source of uncertainty affecting actuarial calculations than mortality itself.[16] However, medical statisticians are likely to be involved in relatively small trials dealing with hundreds, occasionally thousands and rather rarely tens of thousands of patients.

The third point is that trialists and their medical statisticians are often not concerned with representative inference. They know that the group of patients they have recruited into a clinical trial are unlikely to be fully representative of the target population. They may have, for example, a much higher mortality. However, in the clinical trial, this does not matter. They are split into two comparable groups and one is compared with the other. It is comparative inference one is engaged in.

The fourth point is that especially where clinical trials are concerned, prospective data have to be collected. As we have already seen, life-tables tend to be constructed using retrospective data (those who have already died) from different generations. In conducting a clinical trial we follow a 'generation' forward. Unless the prognosis is very poor it can take a while for everybody to die. Indeed, the last patient could possibly die after the medical statistician and quite probably, if it is a trial of a pharmaceutical, after the patent has expired. This makes it practically unattractive to follow all the patients in a trial until death and the problem then becomes that of deciding on the effect of a treatment on mortality without having studied everyone.

Out of all proportion

Nevertheless, without observing deaths you cannot decide on the effect of treatments on mortality so that it is deaths you have to collect. If, however, not everybody dies, and your trial is in any case small, you end up with even less information than one might suppose is the case simply by looking at

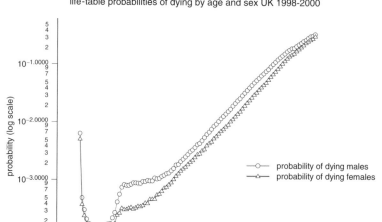

Figure 7.3 Probability of dying before next birthday by age and sex for the United Kingdom 1998–2000. Source Government Actuary's Department. Note vertical scale is logarithmic.

the number of patients. Now suppose that you wish to study the effect of a new treatment on survival of patients who have had a myocardial infarction. Patients are randomly assigned to the new treatment or the control treatment. But how shall you summarise the difference between the two groups? Figure 7.3 shows the problem. This is not of a clinical trial but concerns the example of life expectancy in the United Kingdom based on the Government Actuary's Department for 1998–2000. The graph shows qx (our life-table approximation of the hazard rate) for males and females based on three years of data. A logarithmic scale has been used for the probability of dying.

What is noticeable is that there is a huge variation in the probability of dying over the various age-ranges. The situation seems difficult to summarise. However, what is also striking is that the probability of dying is higher at each age for males than for females. This is not so easily seen on the graph, especially at the lower ages. However, we can remember a lesson we learned when looking at Arbuthnot's birth data. If you are interested in differences and ratios, and ratios *are* what I am interested in here, then you should plot these. Figure 7.4 gives the ratio of the life-table

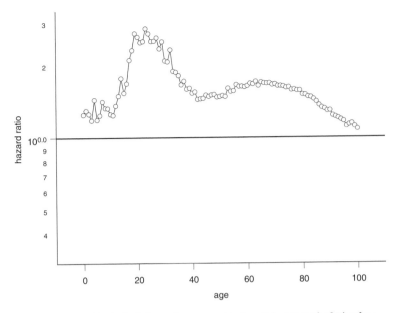

Figure 7.4 Hazard ratio for being male compared to female by age. United Kingdom 1998–2000. Note vertical scale is logarithmic.

probability of dying for males compared to females. As we have already discussed, this probability is very nearly the hazard rate. What the diagram plots is the hazard ratio.

As with the probabilities, the hazard ratio has been plotted on a logarithmic scale. The horizontal line is at a ratio of 1, which has a logarithm of zero. Since the logarithm of a ratio is the difference in logarithms, what has been plotted is the difference between the two curves on the first plot. We can now see quite clearly that the probability of dying is always higher for males than for females. In addition, however, if we study the age range 40 to 75, we shall find that in this range the hazard ratio varies very little and is close to 1.5. To emphasise this, Figure 7.5 plots the hazard ratio for the age range in question.

Now suppose that we are asked to summarise the mortality of males. This is very difficult since the picture is extremely complex. On the other hand, if asked to summarise the difference it makes to mortality being male rather than female in the age range 40 to 75, then this is very easy. The effect is to multiply the hazard rate by about 1.5.

There is one particular circumstance under which this sort of summary is particularly useful and that is when you are reporting a clinical

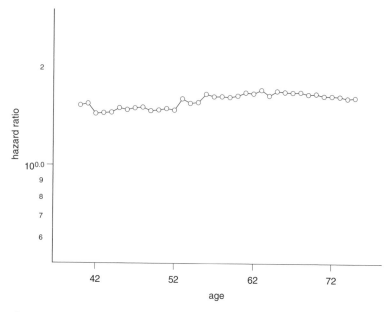

Figure 7.5 Hazard ratio for being male compared to female by age, age 40–75. United Kingdom 1998–2000. Note vertical scale is logarithmic.

trial. There, survival time will not be measured from birth but from the moment the treatment is given. However, unlike when constructing a life-table for the United Kingdom, we will have very few data available to estimate the effect of treatment on each possible length of survival. If we can assume, however, that the effect is approximately proportionate on the hazard scale, which is to say that the hazard ratio will be constant, then we can hope to use data from the whole trial to tell us what this ratio is.

Before Cox published his much-cited work, statisticians were already able to deal with the fact that in a clinical trial not all of the patients will have died. This phenomenon is called censoring. We have to replace an exact value for the years survived with an inexact one; for example, this patient survived at least five years (if still alive after five years at the end of the trial). Statisticians could also include many variables. In a clinical trial, you are measuring survival from the moment treatment is given, or perhaps from the time of infarct, but not from birth, yet the age of the patient, and quite possibly sex and probably some measure of baseline risk and whether the patient is a smoker or not might all plausibly have an effect. You may feel you ought to take account of all these factors in your analysis. Such factors, which are not of direct interest, are usually referred to as covariates and sometimes as nuisance variables. However, in allowing for these factors, statisticians had to use a so-called parametric model. That is to say they had to postulate a particular mathematical form for survival and see how treatment altered it. This was problematic because it was difficult to know what form was appropriate, there might not be a simple form that would do the facts justice and you might have difficulty checking from the data which form was best.

What Cox's paper showed was that the inferences you made did not require precise modelling of the background probability of dying, as long as it was the hazard ratio you were interested in; in fact this probability has very little influence on inferences about the hazard ratio. In other words, it was not necessary to establish accurately what the life-table was for each group in order to make inferences about the differences in mortality on the log-hazard scale. This was its principle innovation. Essentially what Cox had done was bridge the gap between the mathematical modelling approaches that statisticians were used to using in this and other fields and the more empirical life-table approaches of the actuary.

Epilogue

As already indicated, the proportional hazards model has become a huge hit, not only with the statistical community, but also with the medical community. There must be at least 40 books on the methodology of survival analysis, many of whose pages will be devoted to explaining and extending the proportional hazards model and every major statistical package permits you to fit it. However, there are also hundreds of medical application papers published every year that cite it.

The author of the paper, Sir David Cox, has received many honours for this and for his many other contributions to statistics but perhaps the most remarkable and the most poignant testimony to the power of statistics is the Charles F. Kettering prize for cancer. There, in amongst the list of prize-winners since 1979, amongst the citations for the discovery of treatments for testicular cancer and leukaemia, and for various cellular mechanisms of cancer, you will find the following: 1990 Sir David Cox, Ph.D., F.R.S. For the development of the Proportional Hazard Regression Model.[17]

8

A dip in the pool

Meta-analyst: one who thinks that if manure is piled high enough it will smell like roses.

Guernsey McPearson, Drug Development Dictionary

Pearson *père*

Always an elaborately careful worker, a maker of long rows of variables, always realizing the presence of uncontrollable variables, always a vicious assailant of what he considered slackness or lie or pomposity, never too kindly to well-intentioned stupidity, he worked in the laboratories of Koch, of Pasteur, he followed the early statements of Pearson in biometrics ...

Sinclair Lewis, Arrowsmith

It is time we had a closer look at Karl Pearson (1857–1936).[1] He has already appeared a number of times in this book but we have yet to give him the attention he deserves. History has not been particularly kind to him. At the height of his powers he was one of the most famous scientists of the day. He seemed to be the biometrical messiah. Little did he know that he was simply preparing the way for one greater who was to come after him. However, if it was the gospel of Fisher that was to spread, it was Pearson who originally baptised scientists in the biometrical faith. There is no doubt that, at one time, Pearson was *the* man.

Amongst the acolytes who owe their biometrical baptism to Pearson are Major Greenwood, the first Professor of Epidemiology at the London School of Hygiene, and Bradford Hill Greenwood's successor. Both attended his lectures. Student received permission from Guinness to have leave for one year to study with him. When Neyman first came to England it was to work in Pearson's department and, of course, Egon Pearson,

Neyman's collaborator, also received his start in biometrics from his famous father. Even Fisher received a start of sorts from him, since Pearson's idiosyncratic journal, *Biometrika*, was where Fisher's famous paper on the correlation coefficient appeared.

Pearson was a strong believer in heredity and the fact that his father and mother were of pure Yorkshire stock was, in his opinion, sufficient explanation for his character, the purely environmental circumstance of London as his birthplace being largely irrelevant. A capacity for hard work and a capacity for roving into other people's preserves,[2] are what he found in himself. Others would have assigned him obduracy and a tendency to gravitate towards controversy and disputation.

Pearson was actually born Charles but as a young man he fell in love with Germany and changed his name to Karl and this also explains why his son was given the name Egon. Pearson's father was a barrister, Queen's Counsel,[3] and Karl was educated first at University College School and then at Cambridge, which he entered as a scholar in 1875, graduating third wrangler in 1879. Already at Cambridge he displayed the predilection for disputes that was to characterise his scientific life. At his college of King's he succeeded in getting compulsory attendance at chapel abolished, then appeared the following Sunday in his usual place explaining it was the compulsion and not the worship he was rebelling against. However, let the man speak for himself.

> In Cambridge I studied mathematics under Routh, Stokes, Cayley and Clerk Maxwell – but wrote papers on Spinoza. In Heidelberg I studied physics under Quincke, but also metaphysics under Kuno Fischer. In Berlin I studied Roman Law under Bruns and Mommsen but attended the lectures of Du Bois Reymond on Darwinism. Back at Cambridge I worked in the engineering shops but drew up the schedule in Mittel- and Althochdeutsch for the Medieval Languages Tripos. Coming to London, I read in chambers in Lincoln's Inn, drawing up Bills of Sale, and was called to the Bar but varied legal studies by lecturing on Heat at Barnes, on Martin Luther at Hampstead, and on Lasalle and Marx on Sundays at revolutionary clubs round Soho.[4]

Indeed, Pearson was a lifelong socialist who contributed hymns to the *Socialist Song Book* and stuck to his principles by refusing all public honours, including a knighthood when it was offered to him. His interests were extraordinarily wide and varied. The above passage, although clearly a boast, is no *idle* boast, for Pearson never did anything by halves. His statistical contributions included work on frequency distributions, correlation and the theory of sampling. His non-statistical (or at least not exclusively statistical) contributions include work on heredity and eugenics and history, including art history. Although Pearson became an atheist, he wrote a passion play in 1882 and a work of 1887 in German, *Die Fronica: ein Beitrag zur Geschichte des Christusbildes in Mittelalter*, which is an art-historical description of the growth of the Veronica legend in the middle-ages. His works on philosophy and religion include articles on free-thought, on Spinoza, Maimonides, Martin Luther and Meister Eckehart. He also wrote a book on the philosophy of science, *The Grammar of Science*, 1892, which was extremely influential in its day.

As a lifelong socialist, Germanophile and eugenicist the following sentiments are perhaps not entirely surprising.

> The Royal Society Council having passed a resolution that mathematics and biology should not be mixed, *Biometrika* was founded with Galton as consultant and Weldon and myself as joint editors. Buccaneer expeditions in too many fields followed; fights took place on many seas, but whether we had right or wrong, whether we lost or won, we did produce some effect. The climax culminated in Galton's preaching of Eugenics and his foundation of the Eugenics Professorship. Did I say 'culmination'? No, that lies rather in the future, perhaps with Reichskanzler Hitler and his proposals to regenerate the German people. In Germany a vast experiment is in hand, and some of you may live to see its results. If it fails it will not be for want of enthusiasm, but rather because the Germans are only just starting the study of mathematical statistics in the modern sense![5]

Gut feeling

Moving swiftly on, we come to the reason that Pearson is of interest in this chapter.[6] This is not for any of his important contributions to statistical theory, amongst which one would have to cite his development of Galton's theory of correlation and the eponymous Pearson system of frequency curves, still less for his ill-advised observations on the regeneration of the German people and the potential role of mathematical statistics in that task. Our interest lies in what he would have undoubtedly considered a minor contribution to statistics, a paper that appeared in the *British Medical Journal* in 1904 and which described the application of statistical method to the examination of the value of prophylactic inoculation for enteric fever.[7]

Pearson wastes no time in discussing enteric fever and inoculation but launches straight into the important stuff beginning, 'The statistics in question were of two classes: (A) Incidence (B) Mortality Statistics. Under each of these headings the data belonged to two groups: (i) Indian experience; (ii) South African War experience'. He then describes data, which he presents in an appendix, which had been collected by Lieutenant-Colonel R. J. S. Simpson giving numbers of soldiers cross-classified by whether they were inoculated or not and outcome, that is to say whether they became cases or not or whether they died or survived. In what follows we concentrate on cases rather than deaths.

Pearson could use data which Simpson had collected from a number of sources relating to the army in India and the 'South African War', the latter being divided into four further groups: Hospital Staffs, Garrison of Ladysmith, Methuen's Column and a group of three regiments. Each of the five sets of results can be summarised using a so-called two by two or four-fold table. For example, the table for 'Methuen's column' looks like this

	Inoculated	Non-inoculated	Total
Escaped	2509	10 724	13 233
Cases	26	257	283
Total	2535	10 981	13 516

If we transform this table of frequencies into one of probabilities, by dividing the cell values by the column frequencies we get the following results.

	Inoculated	Non-inoculated	Overall
Escaped	0.990	0.977	0.979
Cases	0.010	0.023	0.021
Total	1.0	1.0	1.0

Here, for example, the figure of 0.010 has been obtained by dividing 26 by 2535.

It is clear that inoculation is far from being a perfect prophylactic. Nevertheless, if we are to take these proportions at face value and accept them as probabilities, it would seem that your chances of getting enteric fever were more than twice as high if you were not inoculated than if you were.

However, the number of cases are few and the question then will arise in the statistician's mind, 'is this just a coincidence or does it reflect a genuine effect?'.

Of typhus, tables and the tetrachoric coefficient of correlation

There are several possible approaches, at least one very popular modern one due to Pearson himself, based on his famous chi-square test. Instead, however, he calculates the so-called tetrachoric correlation coefficient. This was typical of the Pearson school of biometrics. During his discovery of regression to the mean as applied to family heights, a topic we covered in Chapter 1, Francis Galton discovered that such data could be fairly well modelled using the so-called bivariate Normal distribution. This is a mathematical device, a sort of probability equation, that can describe two-dimensional data such as for example, heights and weights of a group of patients, or blood pressure at baseline and blood pressure at outcome.

When one has a given variable, such as systolic blood pressure at baseline, one can always standardise it by subtracting the average value, the mean, and dividing by the statistician's measure of spread, the standard deviation, which we encountered in Chapter 5. The net effect of this is that all bivariate Normal distributions are characterised by a single statistic, the so-called correlation coefficient, which we also mentioned in Chapter 5, and, to the extent that this mathematical model applies, the strength of association can be expressed by this single coefficient. Some such scatterplots, with their correlation coefficients are given in Figure 8.1.

Here we imagine we have two standardised variables Y_1 and Y_2. This means that in all cases the mean values of Y_1 and Y_2 are zero and in all cases their standard deviation, which characterises their spread, is 1. If the reader studies the four plots, he or she will see that the spread along each axis is more or less the same in each direction and centred on zero. What differs in the plots is the association between one dimension and another.

The northwest plot is the case where there is no relationship between the two variables. A circular scatter is the consequence. The northeast plot is the case of moderate relationship. In the southwest plot we actually have a moderate inverse relationship: as Y_1 increases Y_2 is reduced. In the final southeast case there is a strong positive relationship or 'correlation', as we

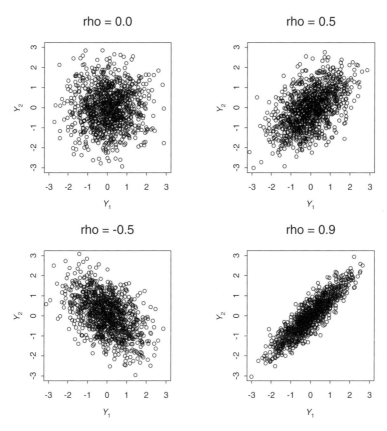

Figure 8.1 Four scatterplots for simulated results from the bivariate standardised Normal for various values of the correlation coefficient, rho.

say. In all cases the correlation coefficient of the distribution from which the results have been simulated is given. It is usual to use the symbol ρ, rho, for this. In general this correlation coefficient has to lie between -1 and 1, the former corresponding to a perfect inverse relationship, the latter to a perfect direct relationship. If there is no relationship, the correlation is zero.

In formalising Galton's work, Pearson came to lay great stress on the correlation coefficient, developing extensively the approaches to estimating it as well as its mathematical theory. Indeed we sometimes refer to the 'Pearson product-moment correlation coefficient'. It was, however, R. A. Fisher who was to provide the eventual culminating theory by establishing how the correlation coefficient might be expected to vary randomly from sample to sample, the first of his papers on this subject appearing in Pearson's *Biometrika*, as we have already explained. At the time of Pearson's paper in the *British Medical Journal*, however, Fisher was still a schoolboy, his work lay in the future and in any case the other methods that Fisher was to inaugurate would eventually dethrone both the correlation coefficient and Pearson from their positions of pre-eminence.

However, for the moment, we will try to follow Pearson as he tries to grind his data through the correlation mill. This seems a bizarre thing to want to do. The bivariate Normal applies to continuous data whereas Pearson's are binary: inoculated or not, escaped or not. Ironically, Pearson is attempting to perform the opposite of what many physicians now do. For example, they take continuous data and dichotomise: systolic BP above 140 mmHg, hypertensive; below 140 mmHg, normotensive, and so forth. This is a fine device for throwing information away using arbitrary distinctions. Pearson goes the other way. He asks the following: suppose that these binary data had been produced by a bivariate Normal distribution, what would it look like?

Figure 8.2 illustrates his idea.[8] Suppose we did have a bivariate standardised Normal distribution with 13 516 observations, this being the number we have from Methuen's column. If we cut it vertically as shown, we end up with approximately the proportions inoculated and not inoculated. If we cut it horizontally we end up with approximately the proportions who escaped and became cases. We can always do this for any bivariate standardised Normal of any shape whatsoever. However, only for a bivariate Normal with a correlation of 0.176 will we get the correct proportion in all four quadrants of the diagram. We have to discover by numerical integration of the bivariate Normal which value of rho produces the desired result.

Actually, either programming this myself or using the statistical packages SYSTAT® or SAS®, I get the value of 0.176. Pearson, whose labours, or the labours of whose human computers, would have been much longer and more tedious, gets 0.19. He also calculates a 'probable error' of 0.026. By adding or subtracting this value from the 'point estimate' we would obtain what in modern parlance are the 50% confidence intervals for the correlation coefficient. These limits are (accepting Pearson's calculations) 0.164 to 0.216. Pearson was a Bayesian, so we might take this as indicating that he felt it was just as likely that the true correlation coefficient lay within this interval as outside it. We must view this with some suspicion.

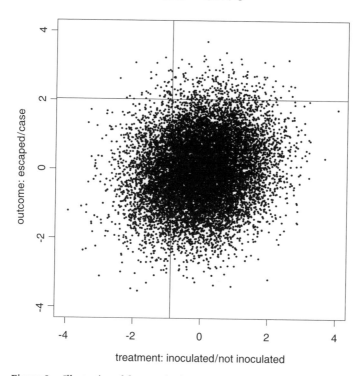

Figure 8.2 Illustration of the tetrachoric correlation coefficient with data simulated to have the characteristics of those from Methuen's column.

As we have already explained, the theory explaining the way that the correlation would vary from sample to sample had not yet been developed by Fisher. When he did develop it, he was to show that the concept of probable error was not usefully attached to the correlation coefficient itself but to a transformation of it. However, Pearson's calculation is otherwise remarkably accurate in this respect. The computer package SAS® gives a *standard* error of 0.0390, which corresponds to a *probable* error[9] of 0.0263.

Many a mickle maks a muckle

Pearson calculates the corresponding statistics for all the data sets that he has. The results for immunity and inoculation are in Table 8.1, the first column of figures being the estimated tetrachoric correlation and the second its probable error.

Table 8.1. *Pearson's 'meta-analysis'.*

Inoculation against enteric fever							
Correlation between immunity and inoculation							
I. Hospital Staffs	...	...	+	0.373	±	0.021
II. Ladysmith Garrison	...	...	+	0.445	±	0.017
III. Methuen's Column	...	...	+	0.191	±	0.026
IV. Single Regiments	...	...	+	0.021	±	0.033
V. Army in India	...	...	+	0.100	±	0.013
Mean value	...	...	+	0.226		

The mean value is the straightforward arithmetic mean obtained by summing the correlations and dividing by five. It is this simple average, perhaps, which has given Pearson the reputation of being the first to perform what we would now refer to as a 'meta-analysis' although, even if one used tetrachoric correlation coefficients, one would not nowadays average them in this way. More weight would be given to those with lower probable errors, although just how much weight is a matter of debate and controversy. Modern meta-analysts would also attach some measure of its reliability to the overall result. What is missing is a probable error for the overall mean. It may well be, however, that Pearson had doubts as to whether any meaningful measure of reliability could be produced under the circumstances.

For example, he remarks that with the exception of IV, the values of the correlations are several times that of their probable errors. 'From this standpoint we might say that they are all significant, but we are at once struck with the extreme irregularity and the low-ness of the values reached.' He seems to be implying that their irregularity is much more than can be explained in terms of pure random variation. In modern parlance this would imply that a so-called random effects model might be appropriate. Later he says, 'Putting on one side, however, the mysterious difference between the 0.445 of Ladysmith and the practically zero result for the single regiments, and assuming that the average correlation is real and 0.23 about, we may doubt whether this is sufficiently large to justify the treatment being adopted as routine'.

This is an interesting observation and is echoed in many modern debates. We would now say that Pearson is judging the results to be 'statistically significant but not clinically relevant'. That is to say he considers the figures to suggest that the apparent benefit of inoculation cannot be attributed to chance but that the effect is so small as to be of doubtful use.

Pearson concludes, 'If it were not presumption for me with no special knowledge whatever on the subject to give an opinion, I should say that the data indicate that a more effective serum or effective method of administration must be found before inoculation ought to become a routine practice in the army'. This is called having your cake and eating it but is pretty typical of the way that statisticians behave. Data are data and as soon as any scientific results are summarised, the statistician will consider that they are fair game. On the other hand, it is always wise to cover your back and, in that respect, suitably prefaced subjunctive statements are always safer. Pearson is not a physician but a statistician. Here he is indulging his, 'capacity for roving into other people's preserves'. There is no need to appeal to Yorkshire ancestry to explain this. The man was a statistician.

More modern meta

How would we analyse Pearson's data today? Almost certainly not by using the tetrachoric coefficient of correlation. A more modern approach to analysis is represented in Figure 8.3. For each of Pearson's five data sets a statistic we encountered in Chapter 6, the so-called odds ratio, has been calculated and is represented by a point. An odds ratio of less than 1 indicates that the attack rate was lower in the inoculated group than in the un-inoculated group. The lines are the so-called 95% confidence intervals and indicate a plausible range for the 'true' odds ratio for that data set.

Also shown are the results of two different meta-analyses. The first, a fixed-effects meta-analysis, uses only the internal evidence of the variability of the results from a given data set to weight them and also to describe the reliability of the result. The second, the random-effects meta-analysis, ascribes to each result a variability that is based not just upon the internal evidence but also upon the extent to which the results vary from one set to another. This latter element of course is common to them all, being the extent to which they all vary, and since this is considerable in this example, the random-effects meta-analysis tends to weight the data sets much more equally and also to express much greater uncertainty about the final result. The final confidence interval is much wider since it has also used the external evidence of the extent to which the results vary.

Of course, the main message from this data set is that there *is* no message or at least not a clear one. It must be conceded that to the extent that the data can be trusted, whether a fixed-effects or random-effects analysis

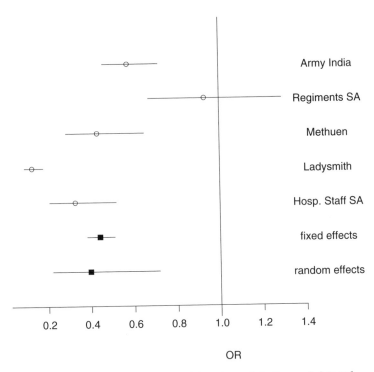

Figure 8.3 Odds ratios (OR) and 95% confidence intervals for Pearson's data and fixed-effects and random-effects meta-analyses.

is used, the confidence interval falls completely below 1, the point at which the odds are equal. This indicates that the result is 'significant': the efficacy of inoculation is supported, or at least the results cannot easily be explained by chance. But they could perhaps be explained by biases. A particular weakness of these data is that they do not come from randomised studies and this means that by current standards we would view the results with extreme suspicion. This is particularly serious because an infectious disease is involved and this, as we shall see in the next chapter, makes results highly variable in a way that is, perhaps, not accurately reflected in the calculated standard errors. Various usual assumptions in the analysis of experiments may not apply and in particular if inoculation was offered to groups of men who were usually together, rather than using true randomisation, then, since cases of infection also tend to cluster, this could make the results much more variable than conventional calculations would allow for.

Meta-analysis is very big business in medicine these days. However, the credit is not due to Pearson, at least not directly. It is time that we looked at two other key figures: a social scientist and a physician.

Gene genie?

In 1965 Gene Glass, [10] who was born in 1940 in Lincoln Nebraska and who had graduated from his local university in German and Mathematics in 1962, obtained a Ph.D. in psychometrics and statistics at the University of Wisconsin. He joined the faculty of University of Illinois in the same year and began to undergo pyschotherapy, with which treatment he continued for eight years. His personal experience of this treatment convinced him of its value. In 1974, when casting around for a theme for a presidential address for the American Educational Research Association, he hit on the idea of a critical examination of a famous analysis of the value, or otherwise, of psychotherapy by the British psychologist Hans Eysenck. [11] In his review Eysenck eliminated all sorts of experiments, for example all those that were unpublished, all those using what he regarded as subjective measures, all those where the objective outcomes differed as to the outcome significant/not significant and finally only admitting a study as demonstrating support for psychotherapy if its outcomes were statistically significant.

Glass set about more or less doing the opposite. He included all studies. In order to be able to pool studies, whatever their outcomes, he expressed them in terms of a standard dimensionless number, the effect size. This is the ratio of the mean difference between treatment groups to the standard deviation of the response. It thus measures the effect as a ratio of the variability of response commonly seen. He did not dichotomise results as significant or not significant but was able to use the effect size as a continuous measure of the strength of the effect. As Glass puts it, 'Looking back on it, I can almost credit Eysenck with the invention of meta-analysis by anti-thesis.' [10]

Finally, he thought of a term for what he had done, calling it 'meta-analysis'. The technique, in particular the phrase, has proved to be an enduring hit. Figure 8.4 shows numbers of citations according to ISI Web of Science year by year from 1981 to 2001. There are 738 in total. This does not, however, do justice to the impact of the term. A search of the same period for the phrases 'meta-analysis', 'meta analysis' or 'metaanalysis' found 14 047.

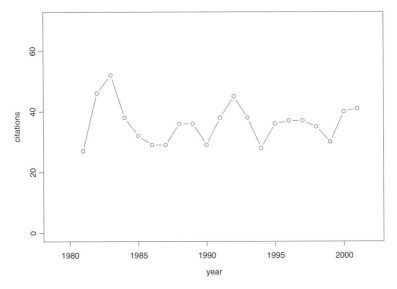

Figure 8.4 Yearly citations of Glass's original meta-analysis paper from 1981 to 2001.

From Cochran to Cochrane

Glass's paper was seminal in sowing an interest in synthesising evidence from separate studies. However, as we have already seen from considering Pearson, this programme was not original. In fact, there are a number of developments in this area since Pearson that one might cite. Three are particularly notable. In 1932, in the fourth edition of his influential book, *Statistical Methods for Research Workers*, originally published in 1925, R. A. Fisher introduced a method for combining *P*-values.[12] Then in 1959, in a paper that has become a citation classic, Mantel and Haenszel[13] provided a methodology for combining four-fold tables of the sort Pearson considered, which, unlike Pearson's approach, is still regularly, indeed increasingly, used. In the meantime, in 1938, Frank Yates, Fisher's chief lieutenant at Rothamsted for many years but by then head of statistics there, together with his assistant William Cochran, devised methods for combining data from different agricultural experiments.[14]

Cochran, although he had already published a paper in mathematical statistics of fundamental importance[15] proving what is now known as 'Cochran's Theorem', had given up his Ph.D. at Cambridge in order to work at Rothamsted. He was eventually to make his name in the theory of sampling, but was also extremely influential in the design and analysis of experiments and wrote a classic on that subject together with the American statistician Gertrude Cox. Indeed, agriculture was not the only field, if one may put it thus, in which he was to consider the value of experiments. He was eventually Chair of the Department of Biostatistics at Johns Hopkins in which capacity he was involved in considering problems of experimenting on patients in addition to those of sampling human populations. In 1976, towards the end of his life, he wrote: 'I have heard this point made recently with regard to medical experiments on seriously ill patients, where there is often a question for the doctor if it is ethical to conduct an experiment, but from the broader view-point a question of whether it is ethical not to conduct the experiment'.[16]

At this point a potential source of confusion must be eliminated. William Gemmell Cochran, the statistician, who was born in Scotland in 1909 and studied at Cambridge, whom we have just been discussing, is not to be confused with Archie Cochrane, the epidemiologist, who was born in Scotland in 1909 and studied at Cambridge. Still less, of course, should either of these gentlemen be confused with Archie Gemmill, the famous Scottish footballer, although it must be conceded that either Cochran or Cochrane, but especially the latter as we shall see, would have been amply qualified to investigate numerically the suggestion that Archie Gemmill's magnificent goal against Holland in the World Cup in Argentina was responsible for a number of heart-attacks amongst the football-viewing Scottish populace.[17]

Having cleared up that little matter we can now proceed.

Of war and Waugh

Archibald Leman Cochrane, 'Archie', was born on 12 January 1909 in Galashiels in the Scottish border country.[18] R. A. Fisher was then during his last year at Harrow before going up to Cambridge, Francis Galton had two more years to live and on his death Karl Pearson would occupy the Chair of Eugenics at University College London that Galton's legacy of £45 000 would endow. Like these three illustrious predecessors, Cochrane was to study at Cambridge; however, his subject was not mathematics, which Pearson and Fisher had read and Galton had dabbled in, but natural sciences. Cochrane obtained a first in both parts of the tripos and after a stint with the International Brigade during the Spanish Civil War qualified medically at University College Hospital London. By that time Pearson was dead and Fisher was occupying Pearson's Chair at UCL. Fisher's office would have been just across the road from the hospital and it is nice to speculate that Archie might have heard the great man lecture on genetics or statistics but I have no evidence that this is so.

Cochrane joined the Royal Army Medical Corps in 1941, by which time the Reichskanzler whom Pearson so admired, had made his 'vast experiment' considerably larger. During the disastrous evacuation of Crete that features in Evelyn Waugh's *Sword of Honour* trilogy, Cochrane was captured by the Germans, a fact, according to his auto-obituary, he liked to blame on Waugh, who was an intelligence officer in that campaign. Cochrane then spent four years as a prisoner of war. Let Cochrane speak.

> The first experience was in the Dulag at Salonika where I spent six months. I was usually the senior medical officer and for a considerable time the only officer and the only doctor. (It was bad enough being a POW, but having me as your doctor was a bit too much.) There were about 20,000 POWs in the camp, of whom a quarter were British. The diet was about 600 calories a day and we all had diarrhoea. . . . Under the best conditions one would have expected an appreciable mortality; there in the *Dulag* I expected hundreds to die of diphtheria alone in the absence of specific therapy. In point of fact there were only four deaths, of which three were due to gunshot wounds inflicted by the Germans. This excellent result had, of course, nothing to do with the therapy they received or my clinical skill . . .
>
> . . . The second experience in POW life was very different. It was at Elsterhost where all the POWs with tuberculosis (most of whom were far advanced) of all nationalities were herded together behind the wire. Conditions were in many ways not too bad. Through Red Cross parcels we had sufficient food . . . We could give our patients bed rest, pneumothorax and pneumoperitoneum . . . We had to attend their funerals and I usually acted as priest . . . I had never heard then of 'randomized controlled trials', but I knew that there was no real evidence that anything we had to offer had any effect on tuberculosis, and I was afraid that I shortened the lives of some of my friends by unnecessary intervention.[19]

In 1946 a Rockefeller fellowship made it possible for him to take the Diploma in Public Health at the London School of Hygiene and Tropical Medicine. Austin Bradford Hill would have been professor of epidemiology at the time. After a brief spell in America Cochrane then joined the Medical Research Council's pneumoconiosis unit. During his ten years in this unit he paid special attention to the problems of measurement and diagnosis, improving both his and general understanding of the associated problems as well as improving the measurements themselves. When the pneumoconiosis unit was transferred from the Medical Research Council to the Coal Board, Cochrane took up a Chair in chest diseases at the Welsh National School of Medicine where he undertook rigorous research into the benefits or otherwise of screening. In 1969 he then became a full-time Medical Research Council director.

In 1971, in consequence of a Rock Carling Fellowship, Cochrane published a slim but influential volume, *Effectiveness and Efficiency, Random Reflections on Health Services*, extracts of which we have already quoted. The summary to that book will perhaps best explain what it was about.

> An investigation into the working of the clinical sector of the NHS strongly suggests that the simplest explanation of the findings is that this sector is subject to a severe inflation with the output rising much less than would be expected from the input . . . It is suggested that the inflation could be controlled by science, in particular by the wide use of randomized controlled trials.

Cochrane was suggesting what at the time was a radical proposal. Scientific method should be applied to managing the National Health Service (NHS). In other words, what were ultimately policy decisions should be based on careful experimentation and scrupulous analysis. If this seems less radical now, this is partly a tribute to Cochrane's influence.

Cochrane died in 1988. As he put it. 'He was a man with severe porphyria who smoked too much and was without consolation of a wife, a religious belief, or a merit award – but he didn't do so badly.'[18]

Meet the Archies

The Cochrane Collaboration is growing so fast that almost anything you say about it is already out of date. According to one source, at the time of writing in May 2002, there were Cochrane centres in 14 countries and 6000 members of the collaboration organised in 50 topic-based collaborative review groups. Yet this was after less than a decade of its existence. 'The Cochrane Centre', in fact which turns out to be the first of many, was opened in October 1992. Its director was Iain Chalmers who had previously been director of the National Perinatal Epidemiology Unit.

Chalmers had read Cochrane's famous little book the year after it was published and, in a foreword to a new edition, explained that it changed his life. It made him determined to seek evidence to justify the way he treated his patients. One consequence of that was an exhaustive review of the literature on the effectiveness of various obstetric interventions. This employed medical meta-analysis to review some of these questions. This confirmed some accepted medical dogma but showed that evidence for the value of other procedures was lacking. The year before he died, Cochrane wrote an introduction to this book in which he suggested that other medical specialties should imitate this approach. He could hardly have imagined the extent to which this would happen.

The business of the Cochrane Collaboration is to answer a criticism of Cochrane's. In 1979 he wrote, 'It is surely a great criticism of our profession that we have not organised a critical summary, by specialty or subspecialty, adapted periodically, of all relevant randomized controlled trials'.[20] The prime purpose of the Collaboration is to provide that summary or, in other words, to provide careful meta-analyses of the available evidence. The Collaboration booklet puts it thus, 'The members of these groups – researchers, health care professionals, consumers, and others – share an interest in generating reliable, up-to-date evidence relevant to the prevention, treatment and rehabilitation of particular health problems or groups of problems. How can stroke and its effects be prevented and treated? What drugs should be used to prevent and treat malaria, tuberculosis and other important infectious diseases? What strategies are effective in preventing brain and spinal cord injury and its consequences, and what rehabilitative measures can help those with residual disabilities?'[21]

The W. C. Fields principle

Q. What is it like growing old Mr Fields?
A. It's better than the alternative.[22]

The Cochrane Collaboration is far from perfect. For example, there is a high prevalence in their community of the obsessive-compulsive disorder dichotomania, the polar opposite of Pearson's syndrome. As we have already seen, Karl Pearson would treat every binary measure as if it were continuous. The Cochrane Collaboration frequently strives to make continuous measures binary, dividing the world into sheep and goats and ignoring the existence of geep and shoats. Nor is the way they handle binary measures once they have them always sensible. Also, their analysis tools are crude. In an attempt to make the actual business of performing a meta-analysis as simple as possible they have relied on methods that are at best limited and at worst misleading.

However, these are minor criticisms and many of the major criticisms of the Cochrane Collaboration and for that matter of meta-analysis in general are misguided. For example, meta-analyses have been criticised because they fail to predict perfectly the results of subsequent clinical trials. This is beside the point. What would have done better? The largest trial to date? Some subjective expert summary? The standard to apply is to consider the alternative. What is the alternative to a careful summary of the evidence? Even if the evidence available is poor, a statistical summary is likely to be better than guesswork.

It has been argued that trials with different protocols cannot be pooled but this is to miss the point again. If the results of trials are utterly dependent upon the specific details of the protocol, then the results are unusable anyway since they depend not so much on the disease and the treatment, but on aspects of design that might have been different. If, faced with a number of different trials, the prescribing physician would be prepared to use any one of them to inform his or her practice, what can be the objection to pooling the results?

Furthermore, what the Cochrane Collaboration has undoubtedly done is push evidence to the front of the debate, by searching for it, by cataloguing it, by discussing it and by publicising it. If some practices of analysis can be improved, as I believe they can, then at least they are available for scrutiny and criticism.

A closely related movement is that of evidence-based medicine. This is particularly associated with developments at McMaster University in Canada and an important instigator and inspiration has been the physician David Sackett. A book which he co-authored says, 'EBM is a process of life-long, self-directed learning in which caring for our own patients creates the need for clinically important information about diagnosis, prognosis, therapy and other clinical and health care issues'.[23]

This involves five steps.

1.   Converting information needs into answerable questions.
2.   Tracking down efficiently the evidence that will answer them.
3.   Critically appraising the evidence.
4.   Applying the results to clinical practice.
5.   Evaluating the performance.

The typical devotees of evidence-based medicine are the anti-thesis of the consultant of yesteryear who diagnosed and treated with hauteur, disdain and patrician infallibility. If they haven't searched the web recently, they know that their medical knowledge will be out of date. They do not prize the clinical freedom to make mistakes but rely instead on combined experience of like-minded colleagues and the data they have painfully amassed to come to potentially fallible but rationally made judgements. This is the great promise that the Cochrane Collaboration is helping to come true. The physician of the future will come in three sexes, male, female and email, and it is the latter, wired for information and trained to use it, who will be killing the least number of patients and saving the most.

Is the evidence-based idea catching?

Let us hope it is. In chapter 1 we quoted Archie Cochrane as follows, 'What other profession encourages publications about its error, and experimental investigations into the effect of their actions? Which magistrate, judge or headmaster has encouraged RCTs [randomised clinical trials] into their 'therapeutic' and 'deterrent' actions?' In his presidential address to the Royal Statistical Society, the well-known Bayesian statistician Adrian Smith, Provost of Queen Mary and Westfield, London, wrote, 'Most of us with rationalist pretensions presumably aspire to live in a society in which decisions about matters of substance with significant potential social or personal implications are taken on the basis of the best available evidence, rather than on the basis of irrelevant evidence or no evidence at all'.[24] He continued, "In particular, there has been a growth of a movement in recent years calling itself 'evidence based medicine', which perhaps has valuable lessons to offer. This movement has its antecedents in the work of people like Archibald Cochrane, who, in the 1970s were concerned at what they saw as the disappointing level of real effectiveness of medical services, and the mismatch between the resources employed and health status outcomes achieved. . . . But what is so special about medicine? . . . Obvious topical examples include education – what does work in the classroom? – and penal policy – what is effective in preventing re-offending?"

Now education and social policy has its own CC, not a Cochrane Collaboration but a Campbell Collaboration, named after the American psychologist Donald Campbell.[25] Who knows, perhaps even in the case of the law these ideas will prove catching? Perhaps even lawyers and judges will come to see the value of evidence. However, our consideration of the law must wait until the chapter after next but in the next chapter we shall look at the statistics of things that *are* catching, whether diseases, religions or ideas. It is time we examined the modelling of infectious processes.

9

The things that bug us*

Faithfully we experiment, assuming
That death is a still undetected virus

Robert Graves, *The Virus*

Infinite variety

There are at least two radically different views of history. One is that all is contingency. 'For the want of a nail the battle was lost . . .', or, as Pascal put it, 'give Cleopatra a shorter nose and you'll change the face of the world'.[1] It is a fine game to identify such incidents. Here is one. Apparently, when the Genovese were looking for a buyer for Corsica, the island was offered to the British. The price was considered too high and it went to the French.[2] But for that we could have had Napoleon as a British soldier and, who knows, roast beef Marengo might have been as British as Yorkshire pudding. The other view is that history is determined by the operation of massive social forces, which render its course more or less predictable. This, of course, was the view of Marx and also of Hari Seldon, mathematician and founder of psychohistory, and the prophet of Isaac Azimov's *Foundation* novels.

On the whole it may be supposed that statisticians belong to the latter camp. As Laplace puts it in a passage we have already cited more than once, 'The phenomena of nature are most often enveloped by so many strange circumstances, and so great a number of disturbing causes mix their influence, that it is very difficult to recognise them. We may arrive at them only by multiplying the observations or the experiences, so that the strange effects finally destroy reciprocally each other, the mean results putting in evidence those phenomena and their divers elements'.[3]

This reciprocal destruction of strange events, however, does not always occur. In this chapter we look at examples where it does not and where a different sort of statistics is necessary. The field is known as stochastic processes and the most important application of it for our purposes is infectious epidemiology.

But we need to look at something simpler to start with. In the word's of Confuseus: *statisticians are always tossing coins but do not own many.* Let us borrow a French sou for a little while.

A penny for his thoughts

The story is that the philosopher, encyclopaedist and mathematician Jean Le Rond D'Alembert (1717–1783) claimed that in two tosses of a coin the probability of getting two heads was one-third.[4] This was based on arguing that the three cases, 'no heads', 'one head' and 'two heads' were equally likely. Nowadays we consider that D'Alembert's solution is wrong. I am *fairly* confident that any reader who undertakes a large series of such pairs of trials (say 600 or more)[5] will find that the proportion of cases in which two heads are obtained is closer to $1/4$ than $1/3$. This is because we regard the four sequences of TT, TH, HT and HH as being equally likely and two heads is thus only one of four cases, not three. We shall refer to this as the 'standard solution'.

Why is the standard solution correct and D'Alembert's wrong? The answer is that D'Alembert's argument *isn't* necessarily wrong, at least not as a matter of logic. It may be shown to be wrong empirically. From the point of view of argument, it depends what you assume. If you assume that the coin is fair and furthermore that the result of the first toss tells you nothing about the probability of the result of the second, then the standard view that you will find in elementary discussions of probability, such as encountered in secondary school, is correct. To obtain the probability of a given sequence of events you multiply the probabilities of each individual event together. Since the coin is fair, the probability of head $= 1/2$. If the result of the first toss tells you nothing about the second, it is still one-half, having obtained a head the first time. Thus the probability of head followed by head is $1/2 \times 1/2 = 1/4$.

However, we saw in Chapter 4 that if we use Laplace's law of succession the result is that in n tosses of a coin each possible number of heads from 0 to n has probability $1/(n + 1)$ of occurring. But in the case under consideration $n = 2$, so that the probability of any number of heads between 0 and

2 is $1/(2 + 1) = {}^{1}/_{3}$. D'Alembert is right after all! The point is that whereas the standard solution is based upon a known fair coin, Laplace's law of succession corresponds to complete ignorance about the probability that a single coin will produce a head.[6]

The declaration of independence

We hold these truths to be self-evident . . .

American Declaration of Independence

If we start with the probability of tossing a coin once, then the two separate arguments that justify the standard solution and D'Alembert's result have this in common. *Given a particular value for the probability, θ, that the coin will come up heads on any given occasion*, both arguments assume that the probability of two heads in two tosses is $\theta \times \theta = \theta^2$. The qualification in italics is important. The difference between them is that the standard solution assumes that $\theta = {}^{1}/_{2}$, whereas Laplace's law of succession assumes that any value for θ between 0 and 1 is equally likely. The standard solution proceeds as follows.

1. If the probability of a single head in one toss of a coin is θ, the probability of two in two tosses is θ^2.
2. The value of θ is ${}^{1}/_{2}$.
3. Therefore the required probability is $({}^{1}/_{2})^2 = {}^{1}/_{4}$.

The law of succession (which would justify D'Alembert's conclusion) proceeds as follows.

1. As before.
2. Let θ vary uniformly between 0 and 1.
3. Mixing all possible probabilities of two heads, θ^2, each corresponding to a given value of θ, each value of which is equally likely, and using the integral calculus, we get a probability of one-third.[6]

In both of these lines of argument let us consider stage 1. If we write A for the event that the first toss comes up heads given a particular value of θ, and B for the event that the second comes up heads and A∩B for the joint event that both of these individual events occur then we have $P(A) = \theta$, $P(B) = \theta$ and $P(A \cap B) = \theta^2$. We thus have

$$P(A \cap B) = P(A)P(B) \tag{9.1}$$

Where an expression like (9.1) is said to apply, then the two events A and B are said to be *independent*. In other words, (9.1) may be taken as a *definition* of independence: the probability of the joint event is the product of the probabilities of the two marginal events.

This *definition* of independence is all that interests the mathematician. Does (9.1) apply? If so events A and B are independent. However, the problem with this from the point of view of the statistician is that we have to have calculated $P(A \cap B)$ to know whether A and B are independent. From the practical point of view this is back to front. The statistician wants to know whether A and B are independent in order to calculate $P(A \cap B)$. The statistician, like the American revolutionaries, wants to *declare* independence in order to proceed.

The way this is done is usually by physical, scientific or practical considerations. One could argue, for example, that the coin does not have a memory. Therefore, what has happened last time should have no effect on the next time. But if the coin has no memory, does it follow that it is tossed by an amnesiac? Suppose that the toss is performed in a particularly uniform way and having tossed the coin we pick it up and return to tossing it in the same uniform way. It is at least conceivable that one of two situations is likely. Either that sequences in which the same side of the coin appears repeatedly are more likely or perhaps that regular alternation is more likely. We shall return to this possibility later. We divert, however, to consider a weaker condition than independence, that of exchangeability.

Rates of exchange

'Indifferent?' he drawled with a slow smile;
'I would be dear, but it's not worth while'

Ambrose Bierce, *The Devil's Dictionary*

Let us revisit our coin-tossing example using Laplace's law of succession but consider the argument as a whole, not just the first stage. In other words we will not condition on a given value of θ, but simply consider what forecasts of the probability of heads an individual would make who used the rule. Remember that to use the rule we imagine the following. A black bead will represent a head and a white bead will represent a tail. Before starting to toss the coin we have one black bead and one white bead in front of us. For every head that we obtain we add a white bead to the pile and for every tail that we obtain we add a black bead. Our probability at any stage that the next toss will show 'head' is the proportion of white beads in the pile and the probability that any toss will show 'tail' is the proportion of black beads. To make it more interesting let us suppose that the coin is tossed three times and we are interested in the probability of getting two heads. Consider three possible sequences: HHT, HTH, THH. How should one calculate?

> Sequence 1: HHT. The law says we have a probability of $1/2$ to start with. Having seen one head the probability of the next head is $2/3$ and having seen two heads in two tosses the probability of one tail is $1/4$. Thus the probability of the sequence HHT is $(1/2)(2/3)(1/4) = 1/12$.
> Sequence 2: HTH. We have $1/2$ to start with. Having seen one head, the probability of tail is $1/3$. Having seen a head and a tail, the probability of a head is $2/4$. Thus the probability of the sequence is $(1/2)(1/3)(2/4) = 1/12$.
> Sequence 3: THH. We again have $1/2$ to start with. Having seen one tail the probability of a head is $1/3$. Having seen a tail and a head, the probability of a head is $2/4$. Thus the probability is $(1/2)(1/3)(2/4) = 1/12$.

The probability of getting two heads in any order is thus $1/12 + 1/12 + 1/12 = 3/12 = 1/4$. However, the point of interest here is that although the overall probability of these three sequences is identical, and although the probability elements for sequences two and three, $1/2, 1/3, 2/4$ are the same, those for sequence 1 are different, although the *product* of the elements is the same. On a given toss, the probability of head or tail changes depending as to what has happened before. We no longer have the condition of *independence*. Thus looked at as a whole, the law of succession does not appear compatible with independence.

It *is* compatible, however, with a weaker condition, that of *exchangeability*, a concept due to the Italian mathematician de Finetti, whom we encountered in Chapter 4. The concept of exchangeability says that given a collection of events, if the probability of any sequence of events is equally likely, the events are exchangeable. If you tell me that you have observed a particular sequence of two heads and one tail and I regard the order in which the heads and tails has occurred as being irrelevant to my assessment of the probability, then these sequences are exchangeable. It often turns out that exchangeability is all that is necessary to be able to make progress in statistical calculation. In fact an assumption of conditional independence[7] will imply exchangeability amongst some events. This is the case with our coin-tossing example. Laplace's law of succession applied to binary events arises as a consequence of two assumptions. First, complete prior ignorance about the probability of a 'success' (for example 'heads'). Second, *given* any value for the probability of success, independence of the consequent successes and failures. These two assumptions operating together do not, interestingly, lead to *unconditional* independence but they do lead to exchangeability.

However, it is at this point that a confession must be made to the reader. This chapter has much in common with a typical Icelandic saga. 'There was a man called Bjarni Siggurdson. He was a great warrior and liked nothing better than to go a-Viking every spring. Every autumn he would return laden with loot. He had a great house near Sognefjord and kept many fighting men. This story is not about him.' This chapter is not about exchangeable events or at least not about exchangeable sequences.[8] In fact it is precisely about those sort of difficult and delicate statistical models in which the order in which events occur is not irrelevant but *does* matter. This is a common feature of infectious disease models and this is what we are going to consider. But who can define shade without light? To understand the difficult world of 'stochastic processes', for this is the term statisticians reserve for this field, we needed to first understand that comparative child's play in which independence or exchangeability can be exploited. Now that we have achieved that understanding we may proceed.

Chain reaction*

We consider a simple example first in which some *small* degree of dependence between events is introduced: a slightly more complicated case involving coins. Suppose we toss our coin in a very regular manner and with great skill, always catching it expertly on the back of the hand. However, we always observe the following procedure. If the coin lands heads up on the hand as we catch it, it is laid heads up on the thumb before tossing it, and if it lands tails up on the hand it is laid tails up on the thumb before tossing it. The regularity of this procedure may make a particular sequence of results likely, particularly if we toss the coin slowly and not particularly far. Persy Diaconis and Joe Keller have shown that a particular threshold of speed and height has to be reached before the toss becomes truly unpredictable.[9]

Suppose, given that this procedure is followed, that Table 9.1 represents the probability of observing a head or tail (as the case may be) given that one has observed a head or tail (as the case may be) on the current toss.

In the language of Markov chains, named after the Russian mathematician Andrei Andreyevich Markov (1856–1922), 'tails' and 'heads' are

Table 9.1. *One-step transition probabilities.*

	Subsequent	
Initial	Tail	Head
Tail	0.91	0.09
Head	0.11	0.89

the *states* of the chain. The table gives the so-called *transition probabilities* of moving from one state to another and is referred to as a *transition matrix*. Here it seems that a repetition of the previous result (for example, tail followed by tail) is much more likely than a switch to the other result (for example, tail followed by head). This does not have to be so. We have already discussed that a regular method of tossing could make an alternating series more likely.

Note that it is a necessary condition of the chain that the probabilities in the row sum to 1. This is because starting from any state, one or other of the possible states (including the starting state) must be reached. It is not necessary, however, for the columns to add to 1. Indeed, in this case they don't. There is a slight excess in favour of switching from heads compared to switching from tails. Similarly, there is a slight excess in probability in remaining on tails, compared to remaining on heads. It can be shown that this slight bias in favour of tails means that if the coin is tossed long enough we will eventually expect to see tails about 55% of the time and that this is true irrespective of how we started tossing the coin. (There is some folklore to the effect that coins are generally heavier on the 'heads' side than on the 'tails' side, so that tails is slightly more likely to end up uppermost.)

For example, suppose we start out tossing with a tail face up. What is the probability that the second subsequent toss will be a tail? There are two ways this can happen. We can get a tail followed by a tail on the second toss, or a head followed by a tail. The probability of the first sequence is $0.91 \times 0.91 = 0.8281$ and of the second is $0.09 \times 0.11 = 0.0099$. Adding the two together we get 0.838. The calculation we have performed corresponds to taking the first row of Table 9.1 and multiplying it by the first column of Table 9.1 entry by entry and adding the results. We can get the three other probabilities using a similar procedure. There being four transition probabilities, this particular process needs to be carried out four times in total, one of which we have already done. In general, take the row

Table 9.2. *Two-step transition probabilities.*

	Subsequent	
Initial	Tail	Head
Tail	0.838	0.162
Head	0.198	0.802

corresponding to the relevant starting position and multiply it into the column corresponding to the relevant final position as described above. Once all the calculations have been carried out, Table 9.2 of 'two-step transition probabilities' results.

Suppose that we regard the probabilities in Table 9.1 as a matrix, and refer to this as $\mathbf{P}^{(1)}$, where the superscript (1) indicates that it represents the one-step transition probability. Similarly the probabilities in Table 9.2 form another matrix that we refer to as $\mathbf{P}^{(2)}$. In that branch of mathematics referred to as matrix algebra, the particular set of operations we performed of multiplying rows into columns is referred to as *matrix multiplication*. Since the same matrix was involved, then, just as we refer to *squaring* a number when we multiply it by itself, so we refer to squaring a matrix. In fact what we have is $\mathbf{P}^{(2)} = \mathbf{P}^{(1)} \times \mathbf{P}^{(1)} = (\mathbf{P}^{(1)})^2$.

Now suppose that we wish to calculate the three-step transition probability matrix. We can use the fact that to get to stage three you have to get to stage two first. If we multiply $\mathbf{P}^{(2)} \times \mathbf{P}^{(1)}$ we will, in fact, get the required probabilities and so we have

$$\mathbf{P}^{(3)} = \mathbf{P}^{(2)} \times \mathbf{P}^{(1)} = \mathbf{P}^{(1)} \times \mathbf{P}^{(1)} \times \mathbf{P}^{(1)} = \left(\mathbf{P}^{(1)}\right)^3.$$

If we take this further and raise $\mathbf{P}^{(1)}$ to yet higher powers we will find that, in this case, as this power increases the result approaches the limit given by Table 9.3, which we shall refer to as $\mathbf{P}^{(\infty)}$.

Note that in the limit, the Markov chain loses its memory. It no longer matters what the result of our first toss is; the transition probability moves towards this position gradually. The situation for our example is illustrated in Figure 9.1 This gives the four transition probabilities as a function of the number of steps. It can be seen that initially the probability of the coin showing the same result on the subsequent toss as on the first is much higher than its showing the opposite result. The value for tail–tail is a little higher than that for head–head. As soon as there are 11 or more

Table 9.3. *Limiting transition probabilities.*

	Subsequent	
Initial	Tail	Head
Tail	0.55	0.45
Head	0.55	0.45

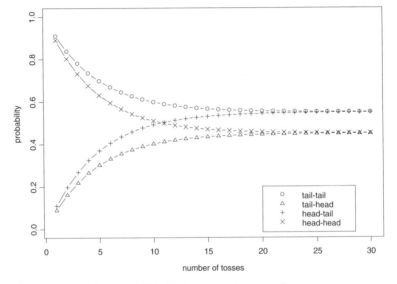

Figure 9.1 Transition probabilities for the coin-tossing example.

steps, however, the probability of a switch to tails from an initial position of heads is actually greater than ending up with heads itself. For example, if you had just seen the coin tossed and it came up heads, it would be safer to bet that it would come up tails 15 tosses into the future than that it would come up heads.

Dodgy geyser or faithful retainer?*

Despite the earlier allusion to Iceland, the geyser in question is not *The Great Geysir* near Haukadalur nor even Strokur nearby, which I have been fortunate enough to observe myself, but Old Faithful in Yellowstone National Park. It seems that Old Faithful has been getting less reliable

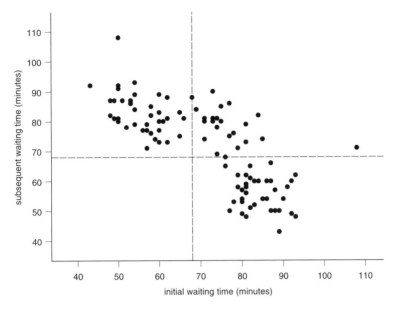

Figure 9.2 Transition probabilities for the Old Faithful data.

with time. However, two statisticians, Azzalini and Bowman, were able to show in 1990 that what seemed to be a rather complex pattern could be *fairly* well explained by a Markov chain.[10] This has no more to do with disease than does tossing of coins but it is a nice and very simple example of a stochastic process so we divert to consider it.

Azzalini and Bowman consider data on the waiting time between eruptions and also on their duration. We shall only consider the former. They have a series of interval measurements lasting two weeks. Figure 9.2 shows data for the first 100 eruptions in their series. The waiting times at a lag of one eruption are plotted against the original data. Thus each point represents the plot of a subsequent waiting time against the one immediately preceding it.

The waiting times are divided into two groups as being long or short, depending upon whether they are greater or less than 68 minutes. This division is illustrated by the vertical and horizontal lines on the graph. It can be seen that whereas a long waiting time may be followed by either a short or long waiting time, a short waiting time is always followed by a long one. Using the full series of data, Azzalini and Bowman show that

Table 9.4. *Old Faithful waiting times.*

Initial	Subsequent	
	Short	Long
Short	0	1
Long	0.536	0.464

the transition matrix is represented by: and that the process is *fairly* well represented by a Markov chain.

Here is the bad news. Although the sort of probabilities represented by Markov chains signify an increase in complexity compared to the simple independent events we considered at the start of this chapter, they *are still not complicated enough*. To give some (weak) flavour as to how complicated models of infectious diseases can become, we shall consider a simple example of a disease model, namely that of a so-called *chain binomial*. However, we have had enough of probability for the moment. Therefore, for historical relief, we consider briefly the career of a medical statistician who is associated with the development of the chain binomial, the confusingly named Major Greenwood.

A Greenwood between two Hills

Major was his christian name and that of his father and grandfather before him and not a military rank.[11] He was born the son of a general practitioner in 1880 in northeast London and, after attending the Merchant Taylor's school, took a medical degree at the London Hospital Medical College, qualifying as a Member of the Royal College of Surgeons and as Licentiate of the Royal College of Physicians. Greenwood is yet another example, in which, as we shall see, this chapter is particularly rich, of a medical man who was also attracted by the fascination of numbers. In fact, Greenwood never practised medicine but he became a very eminent statistician. He worked at first as a demonstrator in physiology under Leonard Hill at the London Hospital, and when he retired from the Chair of Epidemiology and Vital Statistics at the London School of Hygiene and Tropical Medicine (LSHTM) in 1945 was succeeded in that position by Austin Bradford Hill, Leonard's son. Greenwood died in 1949 and, fittingly, it was Bradford Hill who penned his obituary for the Royal Statistical Society.

Greenwood was the first holder of the Chair at the LSHTM to which he was appointed in 1924. In the meantime he had studied statistics at University College London under Karl Pearson. In 1910 he left the London Hospital to take up the post of statistician at the Lister Institute of Preventive Medicine. At about the same time he became a Fellow of the Royal Statistical Society. He was eventually to become its president and win the prestigious Guy Medal both in silver (in 1924) and in gold (1945).

Greenwood had an influential collaboration with George Udny Yule, one of Karl Pearson's lieutenants in the development of correlation. Greenwood worked on research for the Ministry of Munitions during the First World War and together with Yule studied data on repeated accidents amongst munition workers. They developed a theory of accident *proneness*. This is closely related to a hot topic of medical research in the field of survival analysis. However, by a not uncommon process of scientific amnesia, a new term has been invented, and the equivalent of Greenwood's and Yules's *proneness* is now more often referred to as *frailty*.

However, what concerns us here is Greenwood's use of chain binomial models to describe the spread of disease in a closed population. He was not the first to do this. An earlier treatment is due to Pyotr Dimitrievich En'ko (1844–1916), a physician in St. Petersburg who in a paper of 1889 considered the spread of infection in a population divided into infectives and susceptibles.[12] Two American epidemiologists, Lowell Jacob Reed (1886–1966) and Wade Hampton Frost (1888–1938) developed a similar approach in 1928. (This was in unpublished lecture notes.[13]) However, Greenwood's formulation is particularly clear and simple and since Greenwood is an important figure in the history of medical statistics, it is his approach we consider now.

Serial killers*

In a paper of 1931, Greenwood considered what sort of distribution of infected cases one might see in households consisting of a few individuals.[14] Suppose that all individuals are susceptible and that the *serial interval* (the interval between cases of infection) is constant and that the period in which cases are infectious is brief. Accepting 'brief' as a rather imprecise descriptor we might optimistically hope that the common cold, or perhaps measles, fulfils these conditions. These conditions also apply, of course, for diseases in which cases are rapidly removed by death. Suppose that each 'epidemic' starts with a single case or *introduction*, then the

Table 9.5. *Number of cases infected per period.*

Chain	Period			
	1	2	3	Total
A	1	1	1	3
B	1	2		3
C	1	1		2
D	1			1

epidemic in such a household will consist of a series of cases appearing at fixed intervals. If, in a given period, there are no new cases, the epidemic will run out. Taking households of three cases (including the initial case), then the following patterns of infection are possible.

Each sequence, or *chain*, starts with a single introduction so that in period 1 only one individual is infected. In sequence A, this individual infects a second individual in period 2 who then goes on to infect a third in period 3. In sequence B, the introduced case directly infects both of the other individuals. Sequences C and D represent cases where the epidemic does not run a full course: in C only one further individual is infected and in D none are.

Suppose that the probability of infection from one individual to another is θ in a given period and that where more than one individual can be infected, as is the case in period 2, these probabilities are independent. Consider now the probability of chain A. We require that in period 2, one of the two remaining uninfected individuals should be infected and that the other should not. The probability of any named individual being infected in period 2 is θ and the probability of any named individual being uninfected is $(1 - \theta)$. The product of these two is $\theta(1 - \theta)$. Since we have two choices as to which is the infected and which is the uninfected individual, the probability of one infection in period 2 is $2\theta(1 - \theta)$. However, to complete the picture for chain A we now require that the remaining individual be infected and this occurs with probability θ. So the overall probability for this chain is $2\theta(1 - \theta)\theta$ or $2\theta^2(1 - \theta)$.

For chain B, we require both individuals to be infected in stage 2 so that the probability is θ^2. For chain C, the situation in period 2 is the same as for chain A, so that one individual is infected. This probability is, we have already seen, $2\theta(1 - \theta)$. However, we now have to multiply this by the probability that the uninfected individual in period 2 remains uninfected in

Table 9.6. *Probabilities for the various chains given in Table 9.5.*

Chain	Probability	
	Order observed	Order unobserved
A	$2\theta^2(1-\theta)$	$2\theta^2(1-\theta)+\theta^2$
B	θ^2	
C	$2\theta(1-\theta)^2$	$2\theta(1-\theta)^2$
D	$(1-\theta)^2$	$(1-\theta)^2$
Total	1	1

period 3, which probability is $(1-\theta)$. Putting this together, the probability of chain C is $2\theta(1-\theta)^2$. Finally, we have chain D, where we require both individuals to remain uninfected in period 2. This has probability $(1-\theta)^2$. The situation is summarised in Table 9.6.

The second column of the table gives the probabilities that we have already calculated. The third column gives the probabilities that would apply if we only knew the final number of cases infected in the household. This might be the case if we did not observe the epidemic progressing. In that case if we simply observed that three members of the household had become infected, we could not tell whether chain A or B obtained. These two cases have thus to be put together and their probabilities summed.

There is a further point of interest about chains A and B. Although the final number of cases infected is the same, the individual probabilities of these chains are different. This is an important difference to the coin-tossing examples we considered at the beginning. As we showed, whether or not we use the standard solution or Laplace's law of succession to tossing coins, the probability of obtaining a given total number of heads and a given total number of tails is the same in whatever order they are obtained. Here that is not the case. Different chains with the same total have different probabilities.

Minding your 'p' s and 'q' s (and 'n' s and 'u' s)

Chain binomial distributions are very different from ordinary binomial distributions. We first encountered an example of the latter in Chapter 2 when considering Arbuthnot. The ordinary binomial is generally

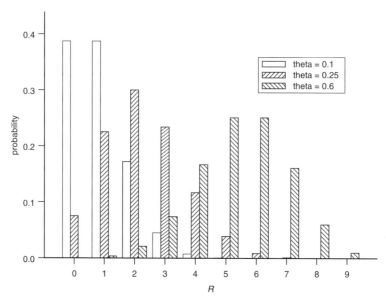

Figure 9.3 Some binomial distributions.

'n shaped', that is to say it has a single peak, a most probable value, either side of which the values are less likely and the probability gradually declines. The exceptions are when the lowest possible value is the most likely, when the highest possible value is the most likely or perhaps when two values are equally likely. The statistical fashion is to use the word *mode* to represent the most frequent or a locally most frequent value so that binomial distributions are referred to as *unimodal*. Figure 9.3 illustrates some ordinary binomial distributions for $n = 9$ and for various values of the probability of success, θ, which illustrate all of these cases.

On the other hand, chain binomials can easily be u-shaped. That is to say that rather than having a peak of probability towards the centre of the distribution they can have a valley instead and hence be *bimodal*. As soon as one has more than three individuals in a household, there is, in fact, more than one type of chain binomial. Greenwood's version was to assume that the probability of a given individual being infected in a particular period was the same as long as at least one other individual was currently infectious. An alternative formulation, due to Reed and Frost, whom we have already mentioned, proposed that each currently infectious individual has an independent probability of infecting each currently susceptible individual. Both of these are illustrated in Figure 9.4. for households of

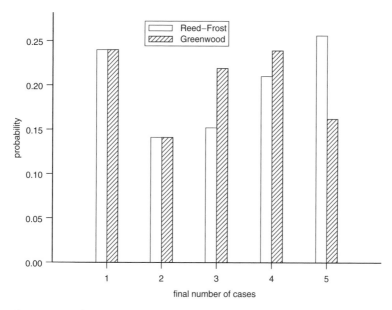

Figure 9.4 Reed–Frost and Greenwood chain binomials for households of size five with one introduction and a transmission probability of 0.3.

size five, assuming a single introduction and for the case where the probability of infection, θ, is 0.3.

It can be seen that the distributions are identical for one final case or two final cases. This is because, with a single introduction, the number of infectious individuals in period 1 is one. Thus although in principle the Reed–Frost formulation has the probability of further infection depending on the *number* of infectious individuals not just, like the Greenwood model, *whether* there are any, this makes no difference when there is only one infectious case. But if the final epidemic is of size one, there can have been no further cases after the first one. Similarly, if the final size of the epidemic is two, there can have been only one further case followed by extinction and so there is no difference between the models. However, epidemics with higher final numbers of infected individuals than two can have had more than one new infectious case in a given period. For such cases the Reed–Frost and Greenwood formulations differ.

However, for either formulation, it is noticeable that it is an intermediate number of cases, in this instance two, that has the lowest probability. This sort of feature is very common in infectious epidemiology but is uncommon elsewhere. A similar phenomenon occurs with more complex models where it turns out that there are particular levels of infectiousness that are pivotal. With values less than this the epidemic tends to die out. With higher values it sweeps through the community and somewhere on the threshold between the two, either event can occur.

We now divert to consider the careers of three scientists, two physicians and a chemist, who contributed to the mathematical modelling of infectious diseases.

Malaria, mathematics and mosquitoes

Sir Ronald Ross (1857–1932) was born in Almora in the foothills of the Himalayas three days after the outbreak of the Indian Mutiny.[15] Ronald was sent to school in England at the age of eight. His father and grandfather before him had served in the Indian Army but by the age of 17 Ross had decided he wanted to be an artist. However, his father wanted him to study medicine and in 1881 he passed his MRCS and LSA examinations having studied at St. Bartholomew's Medical School and he immediately entered the Madras Medical Service as a surgeon.

In 1888 on leave in London for a year he took the Diploma of Public Health and studied bacteriology. From 1890 onwards Ross began a study of malaria and on a second period of leave in London in 1894, he was convinced by Sir Patrick Manson (1844–1922) of the probable truth of the mosquito theory of the spread of malaria. Ross returned to Bombay in April 1895 and spent the next three years working on malaria whenever his duties permitted. In July 1898 Manson was able to announce the results of Ross's work on the life cycle of the plasmodium protozoon, the malaria parasite, at a meeting of the British Medical Association in Edinburgh. By 1900 Ross and others had shown that malaria was transmitted by the bite of the anopheles mosquito.

Ross retired from the Indian Medical Service in 1899 to become first a lecturer and then professor at the Liverpool School of Tropical Medicine. During his time there (until 1913) he organised trips to Sierra Leone, West Africa, Mauritius, Spain, Cyprus and Greece mainly in connection with the prevention of malaria. He was awarded the Nobel Prize for Medicine in 1902. During the First World War Ross became a Consultant to Malaria to the War Office and in 1917 on a mission to Salonika on a malaria survey, the ship he was in was torpedoed. The remainder of his working life was spent in London.

Ross's interests were not confined to Medicine. In the words of John Masefield, 'He was an extraordinary man, for he made himself famous as a poet, and was an eminent mathematician, a clever painter, and a skilled musician'.[16] His Royal Society obituarist, speaking of Ross as a young man, had the following to say. "He was not interested in medicine. During his first six years in India he gave most of his time to mathematics. In his last letter from India when about to embark for home in 1899, he asked the writer 'Can you tell me whether Immunity has been ever studied mathematically?'"

Ross was to supply the theory himself but that story must wait until we have covered the careers of two other scientists.

Big Mac

McKendrick stands in a class by himself.

J. O. Irwin[17]

Anderson Gray McKendrick was born in Glasgow in 1876.[18] Like Austin Bradford Hill after him, McKendrick was the son of a famous physiologist. Like Bradford Hill, his talents led him to apply mathematics to medicine. He graduated in medicine and joined the Indian Medical Service. He was with the army in Somaliland in the campaign against the Mahdi of the Sudan. He also spent a short while studying malaria in Sierra Leone with Ronald Ross.

McKendrick spent many years in India and eventually rose to the rank of Lieutenant Colonel in the Medical Service. He worked in the Pasteur Institute in Kausali in Southern India before becoming a statistical officer with the Government of India in Simla. He returned to the Pasteur Institute as its head. He contracted tropical sprue, a disease that is characterised by inflammation of the lining of the small intestine, diarrhoea and weight loss, and often improves spontaneously on return to temperate climates. McKendrick was sent to Britain to recuperate and during his leave was appointed in 1920 as Superintendent of the Laboratory of the Royal College of Physicians of Edinburgh, a post he held for over 20 years. McKendrick died in retirement in Carrbridge in 1943.

McKendrick was recognised as an expert on rabies. He also studied malaria. Like Greenwood after him, he compared Sweden and Great Britain in terms of mortality. However, as his career progressed he began to take more and more interest in the mathematical modelling of infectious diseases. He is now famous for three contributions in particular. In 1914 he derived equations for a so-called pure birth process and a type of birth-death process (neither of which will concern us here) and also stated some differential equations for a deterministic general epidemic. In a series of papers with W. O. Kermack starting in 1927, that we shall consider in due course, he established equations for the deterministic form of a general epidemic.

The dark threshold

William Ogilvy Kermack (1898–1970) was born the son of a 'postie' in Kirriemuir, a small town in Angus at the foot of Glen Clova, one of the finest Glens in Scotland and one in which I myself have had many a fine hill-walk or ski-tour. His mother died in 1904 and he was mainly brought up by his father's sisters.[19] In 1914, aged 16, Kermack entered Aberdeen University to take a combined MA and BSc course. His study included English, physics, chemistry and mathematics. He left Aberdeen in 1918 with a first-class degree and four prizes, including two in mathematics.

After Aberdeen he had six month's service in the Royal Air Force before going to work with W. H. Perkin junior (son of the discoverer of Aniline) at the Dyson Perrins Laboratory in Oxford. Then, in 1921 Kermack was appointed in charge of the Chemical Section of the Royal College of Physicians Laboratory in Edinburgh. On the evening of Monday 2 June 1924 an experiment on which Kermack was working alone exploded, spraying caustic alkali into his eyes. He spent two months in hospital and was discharged completely blind. He was 26 years old.

There then followed 25 years of extraordinary research output: extraordinary by virtue of its variety as much as because of the handicap from which Kermack suffered. Kermack was primarily a chemist but also had an extremely strong mathematical interest. In that latter field he not only made contributions to modelling infectious diseases, which we shall discuss later, but he collaborated with W. H. MacCrea on four papers, developing an algebra for solving a certain class of differential equation, with MacCrea and Whittaker on geodesics and again with MacCrea on Milne's theory of 'kinematic relativity'. Kermack is not the only example of a blind mathematician: the incomparable Euler, the most prolific mathematician of all time, also worked when blind but at that stage he already had a long career as a mathematician behind him and had been able to prepare for his condition as he knew he was going blind. Kermack didn't begin to publish mathematics until after his accident.

Differential disease[20]*

The reason that Kermack is of interest here, however, is due to his collaboration with McKendrick on the modelling of infectious processes. In a paper of 1927 they consider an epidemic in which initially susceptible individuals become infected and then immune to further infection. The model they use is *deterministic*. That is to say they model rates rather than probabilities. The alternative is, of course, a stochastic model. An epidemic that followed a deterministic model would proceed like clockwork. Of course in practice no epidemic proceeds like clockwork but, nevertheless, such a model can be revealing.

The model is as follows. If the population is of size N at time t and there are x susceptibles, y infectives and z immunes then we have

$$N = x + y + z.$$

Here it is to be understood that x, y, z are not constants but numbers whose value will vary over time, the object of the exercise being to find out exactly how.

Next Kermack and McKendrick set up three differential equations to describe the rate of change of susceptibles, infectives and immunes over time. Using the usual notation in calculus that $\frac{dw}{dt}$ stands for the 'derivative' of some variable w with respect to t and is the instantaneous rate of change of w at time t we may write these as

$$\frac{dx}{dt} = -\beta xy, \tag{9.2}$$

$$\frac{dy}{dt} = \beta xy - \gamma y, \tag{9.3}$$

$$\frac{dz}{dt} = \gamma y. \tag{9.4}$$

Let us look at the last of these three, (9.4), first. This simply says that the rate at which the number of immune individuals grows is directly proportional to the number of infected individuals, the coefficient γ governing the rate. Since it is assumed here that infection eventually grants immunity and that this is the only way it is granted, this is, as a first approximation, a not unreasonable assumption.

The first of the equations, (9.2), is slightly more complex. This says that the rate at which the number of susceptibles changes over time is proportional to two things. First how many susceptibles, x, there are and second how many individuals, y, there are to infect them. Since the number of susceptibles will decline with time, a minus sign is conventionally attached to the rate. If it were not, it would simply mean that the constant of proportionality, β, attached to this equation would be negative. As it is written, it is positive.

We can now see the origin of the second of the two equations. This simply says that the rate at which the number of infectives is growing over time is the number of susceptibles becoming infective minus the number of infectives becoming immune. Since a decrease in susceptibles is an increase in infectives and since an increase in immunes is a decrease in infectives, we simply take the two rates we previously had, change their signs and add them together.

As Kermack and McKendrik note, in a system modelled in this way, a key concept is the relative removal rate $\rho = (\gamma/\beta)$. The numerator of this represents the rate at which infectives become immune and the denominator represents the rate at which susceptibles become infected. It seems intuitively plausible that the virulence of the epidemic will be governed largely by this ratio. In fact we can re-write (9.3) as

$$\frac{dy}{dt} = \beta y(x - \rho). \tag{9.5}$$

Remember, these equations describe the way that the epidemic is changing at any time. Suppose that the epidemic starts at time $t = 0$, when there are x_0 susceptibles. Substituting in (9.5) we see that the rate of change of infectious cases at that time will then be

$$\beta y(x_0 - \rho). \tag{9.6}$$

Now, unless the initial number of susceptibles, x_0, exceeds the relative removal rate, ρ, the term in brackets in (9.6) will be negative and this means that the epidemic will not take off. This is the first part of the celebrated threshold theorem of Kermack and McKendrick. The second part is too complicated to derive here but boils down to this. It turns out that the theory predicts that some susceptibles will escape infection. If the initial number of susceptibles is not much greater than the relative removal rate, then the number that will escape infection is approximately twice the relative removal rate minus the initial number of susceptibles. For example, if the relative removal rate is 900 and the susceptible population is 1000, approximately 800 will escape infection.

The implications of the threshold theorem are important since it implies that if the number of susceptibles drops below the threshold, then an epidemic cannot take off. Thus programmes of immunisation and vaccination can confer a 'herd immunity' provided that uptake is adequate. This in turn raises the possibility of a conflict between ethical and rational behaviour. Since such programmes commonly carry some (very) small risk, your best strategy is not to immunise your child if you can guarantee that everybody else will show civic responsibility. With many parents suspicious (in my view, with little cause) that the measles/mumps/rubella vaccine, MMR, may have serious side-effects, this is currently a very relevant issue.

Most modern epidemiologists regard the 'threshold theorem' as being the work of Kermack and McKendrick. In fact, it was recently realised that many of its elements were anticipated by Ross who included the three equations in several papers he wrote on the mathematics of epidemics. (Two of these were in conjunction with Hilda Phoebe Hudson, a Cambridge educated mathematician who, although bracketed with the seventh wrangler in her year, which is to say amongst the top seven or eight mathematicians, was, due to the Cambridge regulations of the time, unable to get a degree.[21])

Of course, these models are very simplistic. In particular beyond a certain population size it is most implausible that an equation such as (9.2), which describes the rate at which susceptibles become infected, can continue to apply, since it simply means that the larger the population the higher the rate.[22] However, you don't meet everybody in your town or city and if your circle of acquaintances is wide, you must inevitably spend less time with each of them, giving each less opportunity to infect you. However, the equation would predict that in a city of one million susceptibles in which 1000 were infected, the epidemic would be proceeding approximately one million times as fast (in terms of absolute numbers infected per day) as in a village of 1000 persons with one infectious case. Thus the rate per individual would be 1000 times as great. Nevertheless, for the purpose of gaining qualitative insights into epidemics, they are important and, of course, in the time since Kermack and McKendrick mathematicians and statisticians have greatly extended their scope.

One such extension has been to provide a stochastic version of the Kermack and McKendrick model. This was first done in 1949 by the statistician Maurice Bartlett (1910–2002). However, it was not until 1955 that a stochastic version of the threshold theorem was found by Peter Whittle. Here we must leave our very limited historical and mathematical exposé of infectious disease modelling. We conclude this chapter by considering a very curious application of the theory.

Divine disease

Donald Anderson McGavran (1897–1990), the son and grandson of Christian missionaries, was born in Damoh India.[23] In 1910 his family returned to the United States. He studied at Butler University, Yale Divinity School and the College of Mission, Indianapolis and in 1923, together with his wife Mary, sailed to India to take up missionary work on behalf of the United Christian Missionary Society. In 1932, after a period of leave in the USA, he obtained a PhD in education from Columbia University. He returned to India where he remained in various missionary posts until 1954.

During the latter period of his time in India he had begun to write on the subject of church growth. A return to the USA in 1954 was to reinforce this interest. It had been his intention to return to further missionary work in India. Instead the mission sent him to research church growth in various parts of the world. In 1955 he published *Bridges of God* expounding a theory that religious conversion is not just a process that takes place at an individual level but also at a community level. For example, if conversion requires crossing communities it is much less likely to occur. This was followed by a number of other books, including the influential *Understanding Church Growth* (1970) outlining a sociological approach to the subject of Christian conversion. Today there is a community of researchers in this field ranging from those whose motivation is mainly religious to those whose only interest is sociological.

One of the techniques that can be used to study the process of conversion is that of infectious disease modelling. John Hayward of Glamorgan University has applied Kermack–McKendrick models[24] to cover 'epidemics' of conversion such as the Welsh revival of 1904. Here the 'infectives' are believers and the 'susceptibles' are non-believers. If the model is to correspond to the more general form of Kermack and McKendrick, it must be allowed that de-conversion also takes place. In fact, Hayward has applied a number of different models to the phenomena of conversion and revival. Again, the assumption of homogenous mixing is a potential weakness of the general epidemic model since this implies that all members of a church congregation are involved in conversion. If, in fact, conversion is mainly carried out by a minority of enthusiasts a different approach is needed. This situation also occurs in infectious diseases if one has 'super-shedders' – 'typhoid Mary'[25] being the epitome – who are responsible for much larger than average number of infections.

Religion is not the only additional field in which infectious disease modelling can be applied. Computer viruses, the spread of rumours and atomic chain reactions are all areas in which the same sort of mathematics can find application. However, now we must turn from looking at rational laws of infection to examining what happens when irrationality infects the Law and in particular whether there is any hope that statistics can provide a cure.

10

The Law is a ass

Dice, n. Small polka-dotted cubes of ivory, constructed like a lawyer to lie on any side, but commonly on the wrong one.

Ambrose Bierce, The Devil's Dictionary

How much shyster do you want with your quack?

This is a book about 'biostatistics'. It may seem to be stretching matters to include the Law. Surely medical statistics has little to do with legal statistics. What the Dickens is it doing here? We know that statisticians are interfering busybodies but there must be limits. What can be the justification for straying from clinical trials to legal trials, from cases and controls to cases in court?

None at all, were it not for one fact. Lawyers are always interfering with the business of physicians and if the medical profession has decided that evidence is largely a quantitative matter, then the lawyers, in meddling with medicine, are going to have to learn that lesson too. Evidence is far too serious a matter to be left to the legal profession to judge. To paraphrase Archie Cochrane, if we have evidence-based medicine shouldn't we have evidence-based law?

Did you have breast implants 15 years ago? Yes? And did you develop connective tissue disease five years ago. Yes? Well it's as plain as a lawyer's fee that the one caused the other, or at least it is until the medical statisticians become involved. My one appearance in court was in a case of this general type. An unfortunate victim of a traffic accident had subsequently developed multiple sclerosis (MS). Counsel for the plaintiff was arguing

'If the law suppose that,' said Mr Bumble, squeezing his hat emphatically in both hands, 'the law is a ass – a idiot'. *Oliver Twist.*

that subsequence implied consequence.[1] I was retained by the insurers. My opinion was being sought on some studies that had investigated the hypothesis that trauma increases the probability of developing MS. The studies showed no link, were of reasonable quality but rather small. My view was that these studies cast *some* doubt on the hypothesis being put forward. Of course, this is a difficult issue. Proving that something can't cause something is a logical impossibility. Absence of evidence is not evidence of absence. As I put it sometimes, a person acquitted on a charge of child-molesting is not necessarily a good choice of babysitter. Nevertheless, if you take a Bayesian view, then if you have a prior belief that trauma might cause MS and some reasonable studies fail to show this, your posterior belief must be weakened.[2]

The eventual judgement was that the insurance company was not liable for the MS. This was a civil case and only had to be decided on 'the balance of probabilities'. The judge's decision was that the balance of probabilities did not favour the plaintiff's case. This, of course, was a tragedy for the plaintiff. Many of my medical students at UCL would have taken the view that the balance of probabilities was irrelevant; if there was any probability, however unbalanced, the individual should win against the corporation. Indeed, it was my habit in starting the statistics lecture to spend five minutes discussing this week's medical/statistical story. Sometimes they were analogous cases to do with pharmaceuticals, such as for example the Viagra 'story' in *The Big Issue* we considered in Chapter 6. My students would often argue (against me) that the fact that the death rate was no higher than one would expect to see if there were no problem was not the point. There *might* be a problem and that being so the companies should pay. I would then put the following to them. Imagine your situation once you have qualified. If any patient you ever treat in any way whatsoever subsequently develops some problem or other not present when they first come to see you, you are liable, will be sued, will be found against and will have to pay. Is this reasonable? Do you want your career to proceed with this threat constantly hanging over you? Is this ultimately in our interests as taxpayers and potential patients? How much shyster do we want to pay for with our quack?

To return to my court appearance, I myself had reanalysed one of the studies using Poisson regression, coming to essentially the same conclusion as its authors. 'Poisson?' I was asked, 'named after Siméon-Denis Poisson, a French mathematician', I explained, 'originator of the Poisson distribution'. In this, I told an untruth, as we shall see. In my defence I plead ignorance not mendacity. The justice, or otherwise of this plea, the reader will be able to judge for him or herself in due course. However, for the moment, it is not so much the Poisson distribution that interests us, famous and important though it is, but rather Poisson's calculations concerning probability and the Law. Let us meet the man first.

Siméon-Denis Poisson (1781–1840)[3]

Poisson was born on 21 June 1781 in Pithiviers, which is some 80 km south of Paris. His father, who had been a soldier, was a minor official and after the Revolution more or less took over the running of Pithiviers, becoming the biggest fish in the local pond. Poisson *fils* was put out to a nurse whose favourite way of securing him when she popped out to do the messages[4] was to leave him hanging from a nail. Poisson used to attribute his interest in the physics of pendulums to these early experiences.

Possion père decided that his son was to enter the medical profession and he was apprenticed to an uncle who set him to work practising the pricking of veins by working on cabbage leaves with a lancet. Unfortunately, when he eventually graduated to patients, his first case died. Despite the consolation offered by his medical colleagues that this was a very common and unremarkable occurrence, and that he could be perfectly sanguine[5] that subsequence did not imply consequence, this cured him of all medical tendencies, and he gravitated towards physics and mathematics instead. In 1798, Poisson enrolled at the Ecole Polytechnique, where he attracted the attention of his lecturers Laplace and Lagrange. Poisson was a lively and vivacious character and became and remained friends with his two mentors. However, important though he was as a mathematician, he never matched them. Laplace, as we have seen, is a key figure in the history of probability but also made many important contributions to analysis and mechanics. Lagrange, although not of importance in the history of probability, is rated by many to be an even more important mathematician than Laplace.

This gets me on to a hobby-horse of mine and, quite frankly, if I cannot indulge a Shandy-like passion for hobby-horses then there is no fun in writing a book like this. In *The Third Man*, Orson Welles as Harry Lime – in his scurrilous attack on the Swiss, a nation of whom I count myself a member[6] – refers to 500 years of peace in Switzerland having produced nothing more than cuckoo clocks. Italy on the other hand, with, 'warfare, terror, murder, bloodshed', produced Michaelangelo, Leonardo and the Renaissance. There are three things wrong here. First, at the time (1948) Switzerland had had precisely one hundred years of peace not five. Second, cuckoo clocks come from the Black Forest in Germany and not Switzerland, which produces precision watches.[7] Third, the situation regarding cultural achievement looks rather different if, instead of art, you pick mathematics. The Swiss have several important figures but the only truly world-class 'Italians' are Archimedes, who was born in Syracuse and is generally counted a Greek and on whose career Roman warfare, terror, murder and bloodshed had a far from positive effect, and Lagrange, who was born in Turin but is usually counted a Frenchman.[8]

After that red herring, let us return to Poisson.

Poisson was attracted to magnetism, stretched his mind on the theory of elasticity, starred in astronomy and generally counted as one of the foremost mathematicians of his day. However, he has three particular claims to fame in the history of statistics. The first is his work on what we now call the Poisson distribution. It is here that I told my untruth in court. I assumed that Poisson had discovered the distribution named after him. I should have remembered *Stigler's Law of Eponomy* which, you may recall from Chapter 3, says that if a discovery is named after somebody he/she certainly didn't find it. In fact, the Poisson distribution was already known to De Moivre, although not, of course, under that name! De Moivre was a Franglais mathematician,[9] a Huguenot, born 1667 in France, who fled to England in 1685 at the revocation of the Edict of Nantes and died in 1754 on the day he predicted. Apparently he had been sleeping 15 minutes longer every night and predicted, correctly, that he would die on the day he slept 24 hours. (It is left to the reader as an exercise to calculate, bearing in mind that it takes at least three to establish a series, the maximum number of days in advance of the event that he can have issued this prediction.) De Moivre made many significant contributions to mathematics including probability theory, where his work on life-tables as well as on laws of large numbers is extremely important. In fact he can be regarded as the discoverer not only of the Poisson distribution but of the Normal distribution also, despite the fact that this is often attributed to Gauss. However, one way or another, he has slipped between the pages of this book and we cannot take time off to discuss this complex figure further.

Poisson d' Avril[*]

... the Poisson dispensation ruling not only these annihilations no man can run from but also cavalry accidents, blood counts, radioactive decay, number of wars per year...

Thomas Pynchon, *Gravity's Rainbow*

So what exactly is the 'Poisson' distribution? We are not going to make any great use of it, although it is of considerable use in medical statistics. The reader who finds mathematics painful can skip this section and no harm will be done. To satisfy the curious, however, it is a distribution that can be used to describe the occurrence of events over time where the conditions are homogenous. That is to say the propensity for events to occur remains constant over time. Where this is the case, the Poisson distribution can be used to describe the number of events occurring in a given interval.

Before we start, three mathematical facts, at least one of which we have met before. First, when mathematicians multiple together a series of integers descending by steps of one, that is to say create a product of the form $k \times (k-1) \times (k-2) \times \cdots 3 \times 2 \times 1$, they refer to the result as, 'k factorial' and write it $k!$. Thus, for example, $4! = 4 \times 3 \times 2 \times 1 = 24$. By a rather baffling but mathematically coherent and convenient convention, $0! = 1$. Second, if we have an infinite series of the form $1, x, \frac{x^2}{2!}, \frac{x^3}{3!}, \cdots \frac{x^n}{n!} \cdots$ then eventually the terms of this series start getting smaller and its sum is, in fact finite, and is equal to e^x, where

$$e = 1 + 1 + \frac{1}{2!} + \frac{1}{3!} \cdots \frac{1}{n!} \cdots \simeq 2.71828182845904523536028$$

as calculated, very approximately,[10] by the great Swiss mathematician Leonhard Euler (1707–1783), the most prolific of all time, who introduced, in 1728, the symbol e to represent the base of natural logarithms.[11] Logarithms are a device independently proposed by the Scot John Napier (1550–1617) and the Swiss clockmaker and mathematician Joost Burgi (1552–1632), a maker of precision instruments not cuckoo clocks, who would have had, we can be confident, a very poor opinion of Orson Welles had he met him. Third, in general, the reciprocal of a number x raised to a given power n is $\frac{1}{x^n}$ and by convenient and coherent convention this may be written x^{-n}. It thus follows, for example, that $e^{-n} = \frac{1}{e^n}$.

So much for preliminaries. Now for 'Poisson's' distribution. If the expected number of events occurring within a given interval is λ, and the Poisson distribution applies, then the probability of any given number of events k occurring in such an interval, where k can take any integer value from 0 upwards (so for example 0 or 1 or 2 or 3, etc.) is

$$p(k) = \frac{\lambda^k e^{-\lambda}}{k!}.$$

To give a simple example, if we have a factory in which the work force has on average three accidents per month we can calculate the probability of there being exactly four accidents in a given month (say April) as follows. We set $\lambda = 3$, and $k = 4$, calculate $e^{-3} \simeq 0.05$, $3^4 = 81$, $4! = 24$, and put this together to obtain $81 \times 0.05/24 \simeq 0.17$.

Note that this distribution satisfies the minimum condition of a probability distribution, which is that over the values for which it is defined it should sum to 1. We can see that the Poisson distribution does this by noting that if k is set equal successively to its possible values 0, 1, 2, etc. the probabilities take on the values $e^{-\lambda}, \lambda e^{-\lambda}, \frac{\lambda^2}{2!}e^{-\lambda}, \cdots$. Hence the sum of all of these is a sum of the form

$$e^{-\lambda} + \lambda e^{-\lambda} + \frac{\lambda^2}{2!}e^{-\lambda}, \cdots = e^{-\lambda}\left(1 + \lambda + \frac{\lambda^2}{2!}\cdots\right).$$

However, by the third of our rules above, $e^{-\lambda} = \frac{1}{e^{\lambda}}$ and by the second of our rules, the term inside the brackets is e^{λ}. Thus our sum is $\frac{1}{e^{\lambda}} \times e^{\lambda} = 1$, which is as it should be.

We cannot discuss the derivation of the Poisson distribution, nor do more than touch on its properties, but we can make one illustration of a 'self-similarity' property that it has. Let us return to our factory. Suppose that a 'month' refers to four weeks of production and we now ask the following question. What is the probability of there being no accidents in two weeks of production? It seems reasonable that we ought to be able to use the Poisson distribution to establish this. If on average there are three accident per four weeks, then there should be 1.5 accidents on average per two weeks and all we need to do to obtain the probability of no accidents in two weeks is plug $k = 0$ and $\lambda = 1.5$ into our formula. This gives

$$p(0) = \frac{1.5^0 e^{-1.5}}{0!} = e^{-1.5} \simeq 0.223,$$

since any number raised to the power 0 is 1 and since 0! is also 1.

However, one of the beauties of the Poisson distribution is that this result is consistent with another argument I could use and which does not require me to depart from my original 'per month' distribution. I could consider the probability of having a given number of accidents in any four-week period including the two weeks in question and then the probability that they all occur in the *other* two weeks. Thus the ways in which I can get zero accidents in the two weeks in question could also be considered as: no accident in the month, or an accident but it occurs in the other two weeks, or two accidents but they both occur in the other two weeks, or in general, k accidents but they all occur in the other two weeks. In connection with the last of these, let us consider the following problem. In total, over the four weeks, k accidents have occurred. What is the probability that they have all occurred in the 'other' two weeks. For each accident it either has or it has not occurred in the two weeks in question. Since the two times are equal and since I am assuming that the general tendency for accidents is constant over time, the probability for this accident being not in the two weeks in question is $^1/_2$. The probability that all k will occur in the 'other' two weeks is thus $\frac{1}{2} \times \frac{1}{2} \times \cdots \frac{1}{2} = \left(\frac{1}{2}\right)^k$. Now I can put this together with my original Poisson distribution. This tells me that the probability that there will be k accidents in a month is

$$p(k) = \frac{3^k e^{-3}}{k!}.$$

So the probability that there will be k accidents in a month but none in the two weeks in question is:

$$\frac{3^k e^{-3}}{k!} \times \left(\frac{1}{2}\right)^k = \left(\frac{3}{2}\right)^k \frac{e^{-3}}{k!}.$$

However, if these terms are summed over all values of k, that is to say, 0, 1, 2 and so forth, this will be found to be $(1 + \frac{3}{2} + \frac{\left(\frac{3}{2}\right)^2}{2!} \cdots \frac{\left(\frac{3}{2}\right)^k}{k!} \cdots)e^{-3}$. However by the second of our rules, the term in brackets is $e^{\frac{3}{2}}$ so that the result is $e^{\frac{3}{2}} e^{-3} = e^{-\frac{3}{2}} = e^{-1.5}$ as before.

Poisson probabilities, properties and practice

This will not be explained the worse, for setting off, as I generally do, at a little distance from the subject.

Lawrence Sterne, *Tristram Shandy*[12]

The Poisson distribution is the simplest capable of realistically describing the frequency of events over time. The basic necessary assumption is one of homogeneity, which is to say that if we wish to have a look at the way in which occurrences vary, then to employ this particular distribution we have to assume that the general conditions are not changing, and that as

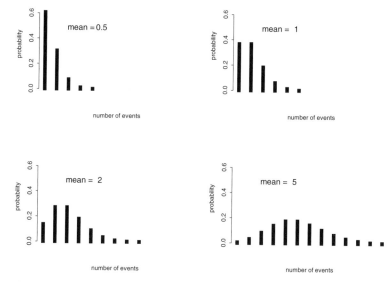

Figure 10.1 Some Poisson distributions.

a consequence the rate, force, tendency, or whatever you wish to call it, of events is not changing.

Figure 10.1 is a graphical representation of four different Poisson distributions, each with a different mean or 'expected' value, λ. It can be seen that for low values of the mean the probability is bunched up towards zero: the likeliest occurrence if the event is rare is that it will not happen. As the expected number of events in a given interval increases, the distribution shifts to the right. In so doing it becomes more spread out. In fact the variance of the Poisson distribution is equal to its mean. The distribution also becomes more symmetrical as the mean increases. Of course, strict symmetry is impossible since the distribution is bounded on the left (you cannot have fewer than no events), but not on the right (there is no limit to the number of occurrences that are possible in theory), although in practice if the mean is low the probability of seeing many occurrences is low. In fact, eventually, as the mean increases the Poisson distribution comes to resemble another famous distribution, much studied by statisticians, the so-called Normal distribution and can be approximated by it.

Another feature of the Poisson distribution, one that turns out to be extremely useful, is that if two or more different types of events are independently distributed, each according to the Poisson distribution, then the sum of these events also has a Poisson distribution. For example, suppose that the number of deaths from circulatory diseases in a given small community followed a Poisson distribution with on average 20 deaths a year. Similarly suppose that deaths from cancer had a Poisson distribution with an expectation of 15 deaths per year. Then the number of deaths from both causes would be approximately Poisson with 35 cases on average per year.[13]

Suppose, for example, we wished to compare the effects of two anti-epileptic treatments on seizure rates in a group of epileptics. We might assume, under a null hypothesis, that the treatments are identical. Of course we wish to investigate the truth of this but we might assume it for the time being. If the treatments are the same, differences between treatments do not exist and so cannot be a source of heterogeneity. However, the patients may very well have quite different seizure rates. This means that it appears that we do not have the homogeneity that we require to employ the Poisson distribution. However, a cunning design might help us here. We might choose to run a cross-over trial in which each patient acts as his or her own control. In such a trial there would be two treatment periods. Half the patients would be given treatment A in the first period followed, perhaps after a suitable washout, by treatment B in a second period. Half would be allocated to B followed by A. Now suppose we compare the total number of seizures for all patients given A with the total number for the same patients given B. The fact that we have fixed the patients means that when we compare the totals, the difference between patients is not a problem. The total is homogenous between one treatment and another. However, the total is the sum of a number of different independent Poisson variables and so is itself a Poisson variable. Hence, we can use the usual theory that applies to the distribution.[14]

There are many potential uses of the Poisson distribution in medical statistics. One is in disease monitoring. If the conditions are stable, the disease is not infectious and is rare within a given population, then the number of cases from year to year should vary approximately according to the Poisson distribution. This helps the epidemiologist to judge whether a given increase in a particular year is consistent with chance variation or in need of some other explanation.

Other fish to fry

We have been digressing somewhat, having left the reader with the promise that Poisson made three important contributions of interest to us and then completely omitting to discuss any but the first, which in any case was not entirely original. His second contribution was to improve the law of large numbers. This is a law that mathematicians have worked on since its first appearance in the work of the great Swiss mathematician, James Bernoulli, whom we mentioned briefly in Chapter 2 when discussing his nephew Daniel. You will no doubt remember Daniel's unpleasant father, John. What we did not mention there was John's important work on the tautochrone, the curve that a descending ball must follow if its time of arrival is to be independent of its point of departure. This has an application in clock-making, that is to say in the making of accurate timepieces, not novelty items in which wooden birds fly out of twin doors on the hour to the accompaniment of strange hooting noises.

The laws of large numbers are ways of relating probabilities to relative frequencies, of stating in what sense it is true that as the number of trials increases the ratio of successes to trials approaches the probability of a success. In James Bernoulli's form this required that the probability of success remained constant from trial to trial. This is a practical disadvantage because one might plausibly believe that hidden causes are changing the probability in unpredictable ways from trial to trial. We may, for example, flip a coin slightly higher or lower or faster or slower and this might translate into different probabilities depending on how we start. Poisson derives a version in which the probabilities may be allowed to vary and shows that the relative frequency approaches the average of the probabilities.

This is not to our purpose here, however. It is the third of Poisson's contributions that we need to consider: an application of probability theory to the composition of juries. This needs a new section.

A Q before P[15]

> The Common Law of England has been laboriously built about a
> mythical figure – the figure of 'The Reasonable Man'
>
> A. P. Herbert

In the 1970s, when I was a student at Exeter University, my friends used to tease me by challenging me to name 100 famous Swiss. Now, if you ask a statistician, 'how's your wife?', he says, 'compared to what?'[16] I pointed out that the population of Switzerland being about one-eighth or one-ninth that of England the equivalent challenge would be to name 800 to 900 famous Englishmen. Furthermore, since my friends were the judge of fame, their own Anglo-Saxon ignorance of matters continental put me at a further disadvantage. To draw a fair comparison we would have to find some Americans (say) and get them to judge these 800 to 900 English names.

However, on returning to England some years later, I discovered that in the folk culture it was Belgians who were regarded as lacking any famous persons. Here they suffer from the same problem, in my opinion, as the Swiss – people often assume that Belgians are either Dutch or French just as the Swiss are judged to be German, French or Italian. So, for example, nobody realises that Rousseau, Le Corbusier and Piaget are Swiss and nobody realises that Jacques Brel, Simenon, Hergé not to mention Johnny Halliday, Plastique Bertrand and The Singing Nun are Belgian. They are all put down as French.

But if I tell you that Adolphe Quetelet (1796–1874) was a famous Belgian statistician[17] you will say, 'Adolphe who? Famous to whom?' Well to Florence Nightingale (1820–1910), amongst others. Quetelet's book of 1869, *Physique Sociale*,[18] was one she studied religiously and annotated heavily.[19] In it Quetelet made extensive use of a now common idea, *l'homme moyen*, the average man: a mean figure when compared to the reasonable man but with rational uses for all that. Quetelet himself had been responsible for introducing the average man to the world of social science in 1835, in a book that attracted a three-part review in the Athanaeum which concluded, 'We consider the appearance of these volumes as forming an epoch in the literary history of civilisation'.[20]

Amongst matters that Quetelet studied in this earlier work were conviction rates in French courts of assize. The figures available to him are given in Table 10.1. The conviction rate for 1827 seems to have been calculated incorrectly and should be 0.611 rather than 0.610. It should also be noted that the average conviction rate as calculated by Quetelet is simply the unweighted mean of the yearly rates. That is to say it is the sum of the six rates divided by six as opposed to the total convicted for the six years divided by the total accused.

From these data Quetelet concluded that the conviction rate was declining. Of course, since the conviction rate in 1830 was lower than that in 1825, in one sense, given that the figures were correct (of which more shortly), this conclusion is obviously correct. However, a more modern analysis of Quetelet's figures would give some support to a conclusion that goes somewhat further than this, namely that the decline is more than can simply be attributed to chance fluctuation. Unfortunately, however, this beautiful hypothesis is slain by an ugly fact.[21] Poisson later analysed

Table 10.1. *Conviction rates in the French courts of assize, 1825–1830.*

Year	Accused	Convicted	Conviction rate
1825	7234	4594	0.635
1826	6988	4348	0.622
1827	6929	4236	0.610
1828	7396	4551	0.615
1829	7373	4475	0.607
1830	6962	4130	0.593
Average	7147	4389	0.6137

Quetelet's data but did not repeat an error that Quetelet had made. The numbers accused and convicted for 1825 were not as reported by Quetelet but were, in fact, 6652 and 4037 and the resulting rate of 0.607 is not much different from that six years later.

Quetelet was also able to obtain data for convictions cross-classified by a number of interesting social factors. This forms the basis for a claim for Quetelet to be regarded as one of the pioneers of social statistical analysis, a form of quantitative sociology. For example, he could show that the conviction rate was much higher for crimes against property (0.655) than for crimes against the person (0.477) but that the sex of the accused made a smaller difference (0.622 for males, 0.576 for females).

J'accuse*[22]

However, when Poisson came to look at such data he made more interesting use of them. In France, during the period analysed by Quetelet, a guilty verdict could be delivered by a simple majority of the 12 jurors; namely, if seven or more found the accused guilty. Was this a good idea? Could some other system have done better? In fact in 1831 the majority was changed from seven to five to eight to four. Poisson had data for the years 1831 to 1833 to add to the (corrected) data that Quetelet had used. These are given in Table 10.2.

Figure 10.2 plots conviction rates over time for the full series of years from 1825 to 1833. There is a definite suggestion of a lower conviction rate in 1831, although there is a recovery in 1832 and 1833. One reason may be that an allowance was introduced in 1832 for extenuating circumstances and this may have increased the willingness of juries to convict because

Table 10.2. *Further conviction rates in the*
French courts of assize.

Year	Accused	Convicted	Conviction rate
1831	7606	4098	0.5388
1832	7555	4448	0.5887
1833	6964	4105	0.5895

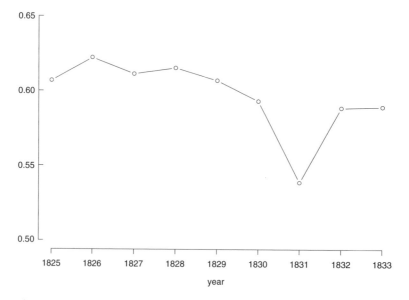

Figure 10.2 Yearly conviction rates in criminal trials in France 1825–1833.

judges were now given more latitude in sentencing.[23] Poisson then uses the conviction rate of 0.5388 for 1831 on the one hand and of 0.6094, which is his average for the period 1825–1830, as enabling him to compare the effect of requiring eight as opposed to seven jurors for a conviction. This gives him two simultaneous equations, permitting him to estimate how the system works.

Poisson supposed that there was a chance κ that the accused was guilty. We can regard this as a probability in advance of the verdict. That is to say, in a Bayesian framework, it is a form of prior probability of guilt that takes no account of the deliberations of the jury. Next he makes two not necessarily very realistic assumptions. The first is that conditional on the true guilt or otherwise of the accused, each juror comes to an independent decision. The second is that the probability of an individual juror coming to a correct verdict is the same whether or not the accused is guilty or innocent. Call this probability θ and suppose that this is identical for every juror. (Poisson also investigates what happens when this is not the case but we shall not be considering this complication.) Now suppose for the moment that the accused is guilty. If m jurors are required to convict, where depending upon the period m will be 7 or 8, then we can calculate the probability of conviction according to the binomial distribution (for details see the footnote[24]). Let us call this $P(\theta, m)$ (this form of notation is just used to show that the probability, P, depends on θ and m). The corresponding probability of conviction when the accused is innocent is then $P(1 - \theta, m)$ because his model assumes that the probability of an individual juror coming to a correct judgement is θ, whether the accused is innocent or guilty, and if innocent then the θ must apply to the judgement of innocence and hence $1 - \theta$ is the probability we have to use for the verdict 'guilty'. Putting this together with the prior probability of guilt or innocence, we can write that the probability of a conviction, which depends on the prior probability of guilt κ, the probability of coming to a correct verdict θ, and the size of majority required m, as

$$r(\kappa, \theta, m) = \kappa P(\theta, m) + (1 - \kappa)P(1 - \theta, m). \tag{10.1}$$

For the case $m = 7$ (10.1) can be set equal to 0.6094 and for the case $m = 8$ (10.1) can be set equal to 0.5388. The two simultaneous equations that result are then solved (numerically) by Poisson to yield $\kappa = 0.6391$, $\theta = 0.7494$. From this he can calculate using Bayes theorem (we spare the reader the details) that with the 7:5 majority system the probability that the accused is guilty given that he or she is convicted is 0.9406.

We now leave our consideration of nineteenth century analyses of the mechanism of justice to look at late twentieth century applications of statistical inference to the evaluation of evidence which will continue, no doubt, to form the basis for research in this century.

The Island Problem*

Sometimes the smallest detail can be telling. For example, John Donne's 'no man is an Island' is obviously true but if one were to write 'no Man is an island' this would be false, as anyone cognisant with the geography of the Irish Sea will surely aver.[25] Clearly such punctuation would be a capital offence but it may not otherwise be clear what this has to do with the matter of this chapter. The answer is, nothing much, except that we are now going to move from considering the application of statistics to the mechanism of the Law and its social aspects, to its application to the evaluation of evidence itself. In that connection there is an interesting type of problem referred to as the 'Island Problem' and in which, it turns out, care in formulation is required, a change in the merest detail leading to a different solution.

'A murder has been committed and there is a known population of possible suspects. The identification evidence, based on information at the scene of the crime, is that the criminal may have a certain characteristic . . . In the Island Problem, the simplest setting for the above analysis, there is a fixed known number $N + 1$ of individuals, one of whom must be the guilty party.'[26] In the classic Island Problem, originally due to Eggleston (1983),[27] the evidence is certain: it is known that the criminal *must* have, rather than simply *may* have, the characteristic in question. The above quotation, however, is taken from a paper by my colleague, Phil Dawid, together with Julia Mortera, in which they consider various versions of the more difficult case with uncertain evidence and offer Bayesian solutions to them.

In what follows let us assume that the crime is a murder, that it has been committed by a murderer acting alone and that the murder leaves $N + 1$ individuals alive on the island. It follows that one individual is the guilty culprit and the remaining N are innocent. If, in the absence of evidence, we regard all individuals as being equally likely to be guilty (or innocent) then all inhabitants of our island have the same prior probability

$$\theta = 1/(N + 1)$$

of being guilty. We also suppose that there is a characteristic C that an innocent individual may have with probability P and we believe that the murderer has this characteristic with probability P^*. In the simplest case, we are certain that the murderer has this characteristic (eye-witness or forensic evidence is taken to be perfectly reliable) so that $P^* = 1$. However, more generally, we can allow P^* to be less than 1, although of course it should be much greater than P. An individual is now arrested, having this characteristic. What is the probability that the individual is guilty?

As Dawid and Mortera show, it turns out that there is no single answer to this. It depends on what else is assumed. They identify six possible cases as follows.

1. *Random suspect.* The individual has been chosen at random and is found to have the characteristic. (Nothing else is known.)

2. *At least one alternative candidate suspect.* Evidence is brought that at least one other individual has the characteristic, C, and so could in principle be a suspect.

3. *Specific alternative candidate suspect.* It is known that some other identified suspect has the characteristic, C.

4. *Full search.* The whole population has been searched and it is found that k have the characteristic, C. One of them has been arbitrarily nominated as the suspect.

5. *Recorded search until one suspect found.* The population has been searched and after exactly k persons have been examined, one is found (the kth individual) who has characteristic C at which point the search stops.

6. *Unrecorded search until one suspect found.* As for case 5 but one has not kept count of the number of individuals examined.

The demonstration of the solution of all six cases is beyond us here, although we shall present a suitable graphical illustration of the results in due course. However, we can (just about) demonstrate the solution of case 1. In what follows we shall let G stand for, 'the suspect is guilty', I stand for 'the suspect is innocent', and, in a double usage that would shock a true mathematician, C for 'the suspect has characteristic C'. As we have done elsewhere in the book we let the symbol $\cap$ stand for 'and'. Thus $G \cap C$ stands for, 'the suspect is guilty and has characteristic C'. Prior to seeing the evidence, the probability that the individual chosen is guilty is, as we have already explained, $1/(N+1)$. *Given* that the individual is guilty the probability that the individual has the characteristic C is P^*. The probability of guilt and characteristic is the product of these two

$$P(G \cap C) = \frac{P^*}{N+1}. \qquad (10.2)$$

On the other hand the prior probability that the individual is innocent is obviously one minus the probability of guilt and is thus $N/N+1$. Given innocence the probability that the individual possesses C is P. Hence the probability that the individual is innocent but possessing the characteristic is the product of these two and is

$$P(I \cap C) = \frac{NP}{N+1} \qquad (10.3)$$

Now of course, in practice we can never know which of these two cases obtain. All that we could ever observe is that the individual has the

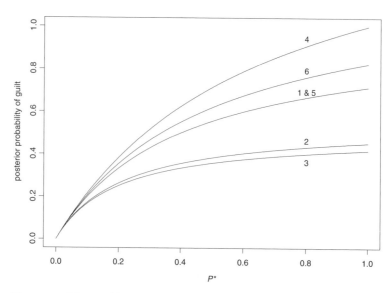

Figure 10.3 (After Dawid and Mortera.) Posterior probability of guilt for the six cases of the Island problem as a function of P^* with $N = 100$ and $P = 0.004$. Where the solution involves k, this is assumed to be 1.

characteristic C. Now an individual chosen at random who has the characteristic C is either guilty or is innocent. Thus we may add together (10.2) and (10.3) to obtain

$$P(C) = P(G \cap C) + P(I \cap C) = \frac{P^*}{N+1} + \frac{NP}{N+1} = \frac{P^* + NP}{N+1}. \qquad (10.4)$$

Having observed that an individual has characteristic C, (10.4) is the factor by which, according to Bayes theorem, we have to re-scale (10.2) in order to obtain the posterior probability of guilt. In other words, we have to divide (10.2) by (10.4). If we do this, we obtain

$$P(G|C) = \frac{P^*}{P^* + NP}. \qquad (10.5)$$

This is the simplest of the cases. The others are more complicated. However, to allay the reader's alarm, we shall repeat our promise. We have no intention of deriving these. Instead, in Figure 10.3, we present some illustrative results given by Dawid and Mortera.

In this example, it is assumed that $P = 0.004$. In advance of any search it is assumed that the chance that a randomly chosen innocent person would have the characteristic in question is 0.004. (The search itself may reveal the proportion on the 'island' to be different.) $N = 100$, which corresponds to a closed population of 100 innocents and one guilty person. For the cases where the value of k is also needed this is assumed to be equal to 1. Figure 10.2 then plots five curves for the posterior probability of guilt as a function of P^*, the probability that the murderer has the characteristic C. (Five curves only are presented, since here case 5 is the same as case 1. This is because $k = 1$ implies that as soon as we started our search we found an individual with the characteristic and this is equivalent to having pulled an individual out at random and finding that the characteristic was possessed.)

As plain as a pikestaff, or as trivial as a truncheon?*

Figure 10.3 illustrates a number of interesting features. Note that as P^* approaches 1 we approach 'certain evidence', i.e. we approach the position where we know that the murderer has the characteristic in question. However, only for case 4, which corresponds to a full search, does this translate into a posterior probability of guilt for the suspect of 1. This is because only in this case can we be sure that no other individual has the characteristic in question. Even with certain evidence, case 1 only yields a posterior probability of guilt of about 0.71. This may seem surprising but can be made intuitively more reasonable if we consider the following (very rough) argument. Suppose that there were one other person apart from the 'suspect' who was known to have the characteristic. If possession of the characteristic were the only grounds for suspicion, it would then be unreasonable to assign a probability of more than one-half to the guilt of the suspect in question. However, in case 1 we have not searched the population and we believe that there is a 0.004 chance that any individual may have the characteristic in question. The *expected* number of individuals amongst the further 100 with the characteristic is therefore $0.004 \times 100 = 0.4$. If we include the suspect this makes a total expected number of 1.4 and $^1/_{1.4}$ is 0.71. In other words because we are far from confident that there is no further individual with the characteristic we can be far from confident that the suspect is guilty.

The most baffling feature, perhaps, is that there is a difference between case 2 (at least one alternative candidate suspect) and case 3 (specific alternative candidate suspect). This a 'paradox' to which the great Bayesian statistician, Dennis Lindley, first drew attention.[28] We shall refer to this as Lindley's legal paradox. Why does it arise? It really has to do with differences between the number of alternative suspects we expect in the two cases. In what follows again consider the case where we are certain that the murderer has the characteristic so that $P^* = 1$.

In case 3 we know who the particular further suspect is. We know nothing about the remaining 99 but a probability of 0.004 means that we 'expect' $0.004 \times 99 = 0.396$ further potential suspects. This makes a total of 1.396 further potential suspects and 2.396 including our 'prime' suspect. The ratio of 1 to 2.396 is 0.417. The argument when we know that there is at least one further potential suspect is more complicated and for the details the reader must consult the footnote.[29] However, it turns out that we need to take the probability of 0.004 and re-scale it by the probability of having at least one case, which is one minus the probability of having no suspects, which in turn is $(1 - 0.004)^{100} \simeq 0.67$. Thus the probability of having at least one suspect is $1 - 0.67 = 0.33$ and the probability of any individual being a potential suspect is now $0.004/0.33 = 0.012$. Since we have 100 persons in total, the expected number of potential suspects with the characteristic in question is $0.012 \times 100 = 1.2$. If we include our original 'prime' suspect this makes 2.2 and our posterior probability is $1/2.2 = 0.45$, which is higher than before.

The preceding example will have served to show that the interpretation of evidence can be a delicate matter. In fact, Lindley's legal paradox is so subtle that it can shock even a seasoned statistician like me. I have no intuition for it and have no alternative but to calculate. This despite the fact that it is very closely related to the paradox *a familiar familial fallacy*, which we included as our first example in Chapter 1. There it turns out that the probability that Mr Brown's other child is a boy is only one-third if we are told he has at least one boy, but is one-half if we are told that the eldest child is a boy.

However, to help our intuition, and to wind up this difficult section, we consider the very simple case where $N = 2$, so that on our island, apart from our suspect, there are two further individuals whom we suppose to be called Smith and Jones. Suppose that the probability of any one of these having the characteristic C is $\frac{1}{2}$. Then the combinations in Table 10.3 have equal probability.

A tick ✔ denotes presence of the characteristic and a cross × the absence. If I tell you that at least one of Smith and Jones has the characteristic then either case 2, 3 or 4 applies. The average number of ticks for these cases is $(1 + 1 + 2)/3 = 4/3$. On the other hand, if I tell you that Smith has the characteristic, then either case 3 or case 4 obtains and the average is

Table 10.3. *Three man island. Possible distribution of further characteristics.*

	Case			
	1	2	3	4
Smith	✗	✗	✔	✔
Jones	✗	✔	✗	✔

$(1 + 2)/2 = {}^3/_2$. The two figures are different. Amazing as it may seem, if I tell you that Smith has the characteristic but I do not know about Jones, then the expected number of persons with the characteristic is more than if I tell you that at least one of Smith and Jones has the characteristic. This, of course, must translate into different probabilities of guilt for a third individual, Brown (say), who is our suspect.

With the Island Problem we have illustrated the relevance of statistics to judging evidence. With Quetelet and Poisson we looked at the statistics of judgements based on evidence. It is time that we looked at statistics *as* evidence. The story that follows is a judgement on the legal process.

Dow Corning goes bust

I am occasionally asked by lawyers why the New England Journal of Medicine *does not publish studies 'on the other side', a concept that has no meaning in medical research . . . Yet science in the courtroom, no matter how inadequate, has great impact on people's lives and fortunes.*

Marcia Angell[30]

In 1961 a Houston surgeon called Frank Gerow visited Dow Corning to propose a collaboration to develop a silicone breast implant. He inserted the first implant the following year. It has been estimated that by the end of the 1970s and carrying on into the 1990s between 100 000 and 150 000 breast augmentations were being performed per year in the USA. The vast majority of these involved silicone implants. However, the technology had started in an era in which regulation was less stringent than now. It is true that in the wake of the thalidomide disaster, a key piece of legislation affecting pharmaceuticals (the Kefauver–Harris amendment) had been passed in the same year, 1962, that Gerow used the first silicone implant but the cultural change that this would engender was still in its infancy. In fact, implants and medical devices in general were not subject to the same legislation as pharmaceuticals. Implants were assumed to be safe, the use of silicone in the human body for medical purposes predated by many years its use in breast implants, but little in the way of scientific research into their safety had been carried out. By 1970, however, regulators were beginning to cast a cold and sceptical eye over the devices market. A study group headed by Theodore Cooper of the National Institutes of Health had compiled a list of some 10 000 injuries and over 700 deaths in which medical devices, from inter-uterine devices to pace-makers, were allegedly implicated. In 1976, the Medical Devices Amendments gave the Food and Drug Administration (FDA) new powers to regulate devices.

In 1984, a jury in San Francisco found that Maria Stern's auto-immune disease had been caused by her breast implants. Compensatory damages of $211 000 were awarded to her to which $1.5 million of punitive damages were added. In 1991 another lawsuit in San Francisco awarded Mariann Hopkins $7.3 million, her connective tissue disease being found to have been caused by ruptured silicone breast implants. In 1992, David Kessler – commissioner of the Food and Drug Administration of the USA, irritated by the failure of manufacturers to undertake the necessary research – banned breast implants filled with silicone gel. This was the signal for a frenzy of litigation and within a few months many thousands of lawsuits had been filed. In May 1995, facing 20 000 individual lawsuits and more than 400 000 claims, Dow Corning filed for bankruptcy. Breast implants had finally gone bust.

It was at this point, however, that epidemiologists and medical statisticians began to take an interest. Not, of course, the same sort of interest that the lawyers were taking. Billions of dollars were on their way from the manufacturers to their former customers but not all of them were to arrive at that destination. Lawyers were taking up to 40% of the awards in fees and of course there were expert witnesses and thus a fair amount of it was making its way to the medical profession. You can't award damages without damage and if it is damages to the body you are looking for, a physician is needed. Nevertheless, statisticians and epidemiologists have to make a living too and it would be pointless to pretend that they are always neutral. If there is a medical story on the go and it has a high profile, it does your career no harm to get involved.

But let's not overstate the problem of doing some valid statistical analysis. If it is an egregious error to suggest that scientists act without motive of personal gain, it is also a serious mistake to forget science's self-correcting tendency. Your success as a lawyer is judged by the cases you win, not by whether you win the truth. This is an inevitable consequence of the adversarial system. Not so for the scientist. Posterity is a vicious crocodile and you can't forget the ticking of its clock. Whatever you say will be taken down and used in evidence against you. Arguments that seemed good on the spur of the moment will appear in the record and will be looked at again and again and again. There is every motivation as a statistician to get it right. Also as a statistician you have an utter contempt for the post hoc fallacy and those who either exploit it or are duped by it. This frees your mind of lawyer's cant. There is only one thing that matters. What do the figures show?

Nobody ever pretended that breast implants were good-luck charms. They can't help you win the lottery. They won't protect you against lightning strikes. They don't prevent your house from being destroyed by earthquakes. They won't stop you getting lung cancer and you shouldn't regard them as a license to smoke. They weren't designed to protect you against getting connective tissue diseases. That being so, given that lots of women have had breast implants, some of them are going to get connective tissue disease. In the same way, every year a very great number of people who have at one time in the past consulted a lawyer when still in good health, die of heart disease. This does not mean that lawyers are to blame for the heart attacks, although the odd client must expire on receiving the bill.

So what is the key? Since women without breast implants get connective tissue disease we need to know whether the rate at which this occurs in women with breast implants is higher or lower than in women without implants. In the years following Kessler's ban, statisticians and epidemiologists began to do the studies that Dow-Corning should have initiated in the first place. In fact, the Dow-Corning story was to break new ground legally. In 1996 Sam C. Pointer Jr., a US District Court Chief Judge, gave a panel of four scientists, a rheumatologist, a toxicologist, an immunologist and an epidemiologist the task of deciding whether there were any grounds, based on existing research, for concluding that silicone breast implants caused or exacerbated either connective tissue disease or the various auto-immune diseases with which it had been claimed they were associated.

The panel published their conclusions in November 2001,[31] although the meta-analyes on which these were based had been published the year before.[32] They pointed out right away the fallacy that had been swallowed by juries, cautioning, 'If the prevalence of rheumatoid arthritis (RA) is 1% and 1 million women have received breast implants, then ~10,000 of these women can be expected to have RA regardless of the presence of the disease'.[33]

Figure 10.4 shows a meta-analysis, of the sort we encountered in Chapter 8, of one of the diseases it was claimed breast implants could cause, rheumatoid arthritis.[34] The panel identified eight controlled studies that could be included in the meta-analysis. Four of these were cohort studies and four were case–control studies. The plot shows point estimates for relative risk (RR) and associated confidence intervals for the eight studies. The scale of the plot is logarithmic since a relative risk of 0.5 is equivalent to one of 2. (To understand this suppose that we compare two treatments A and B. If A has half the risk of B then B has twice the risk of A and since it is arbitrary which way round we choose to look at things, these are equivalent.)

In this case the RR is the estimate of risk of a woman who had implants getting rheumatoid arthritis as a ratio of the risk for a woman who did not have implants. Hence, a value of more than one in a given study shows that

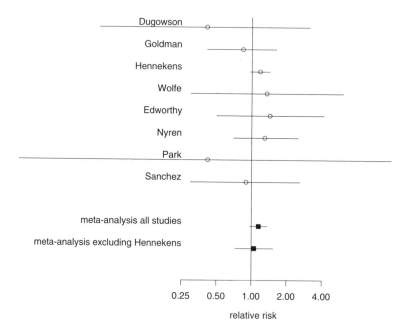

Figure 10.4 Meta-analysis (based on Hulka[35]).

the rate was higher amongst women with implants. Where the value is less than one then the rate was lower amongst women with implants. For each study the so-called point estimate, the best guess as to the true value, is indicated by an open circle. Some of the studies were very small, for example that of Park, and these have very wide confidence intervals. These intervals are indicated by the horizontal lines and give a range of plausible values. For every study the interval covers one, indicating that the range of plausible values includes a relative risk of one or, to put it another way, that the result is not 'significant' at the 5% level.

Also shown are the results of two meta-analyses. The first one includes the study by Hennekens, the second does not. Not only is the study by Hennekens[36] the largest, yielding the most 'precise' estimate, but it is the only one relying on self-reported illness. Since it dates from an era after the implants story broke, the suspicion is that there may be some sort of 'nocebo' effect where by women who have implants are more likely to report disease. Neither of these two confidence intervals excludes one and so the results are not 'significant'. Of course, the confidence intervals do not completely exclude a modest adverse effect of breast implants but they exclude any dramatic relative risk.

However, this is only one of the diseases studied and for some of the others the effect is significant (but very moderate) if the Hennekens study is included. For example for all connective tissue diseases combined, the confidence intervals for the relative risks are 1.01 to 1.28 including the Hennekens study with a point estimate of 1.14 (in other words a 14% elevation of risk) and 0.62 to 1.04 with a point estimate of 0.80 (a 20% reduction in risk) excluding that study.

The problem of Hermione

> There may be in the cup.
> A spider steeped, and one may drink, depart
> And yet partake no venom for his knowledge
> Is not infected; but if one present
> The abhorr'd ingredient to his eye, make known
> How he hath drunk, he cracks his gorge, his sides
> With violent hefts
>
> Shakespeare, *The Winter's Tale*[37]

Where does this leave us? In the koan at the end of Chapter 4 we encountered a problem I referred to as, 'the jealous husband's dilemma'. How do you prove your wife is faithful? The puzzle of proving a wife faithful is precisely the one that Shakespeare has to solve in *The Winter's Tale*. Although there have been some revisionist interpretations of this play inviting us to believe Leontes that Hermione is guilty, I am convinced that we are *meant* to interpret this as a tale of groundless jealous paranoia and since I am not a structuralist I regard authorial intentions as important.[38] So what is the dramatic problem? Shakespeare has to secure a triple 'conviction'. Through the play he has to convince any lingering doubters in the audience that Hermione is innocent. Within the play he has to convince Leontes of her innocence. Finally, again through the play he has to convince the audience that Leontes is convinced. How can he do this? There is no evidence he can bring. He resorts to an oracle: the oracle of Delphos. The oracle is delivered sealed and then opened: Hermione is innocent and a prophetic threat is delivered, '*the king shall live without an heir unless that which is lost is found*'.[39] Leontes disbelieves the message but then immediately is brought news that his son has died, thus delivering both proof of the oracle's prophetic power and a judgement on him. A broken man, Leontes realises his folly and repents.

To convince those who have already decided that breast implants are poison would need something comparable. Unfortunately there can be no such denouement to the breast implants story. It has gone beyond a matter of evidence. Many epidemiologists would feel unhappy about claiming any causal relationship between breast implants and connective tissue disease. Even including a debatable study, that of Hennekens, the effect is so modest that one could not be confident it was not due to bias. Furthermore when the study with the most plausible source of bias is excluded the effect disappears.

On the other hand, well before the statisticians and epidemiologists got involved the judicial juggernaut had already developed its billion-dollar momentum. It wasn't going to be stopped by mere statistics. As Howard Jacobson puts it describing denial of guilt in another context, 'A rebuttal was reasonable and understandable, but it was no more than a response; it came second'.[40] Or, to quote Mandy Rice-Davies on being told that Lord Astor had denied her allegations, 'He would wouldn't he?'. All those who had already made their minds up about the truth of this story were not going to have their minds changed by evidence, still less by lack of evidence, which is the most an accused company can hope for under such circumstances. After all Dow-Corning would say there was no problem, wouldn't they?

Oh, and by the way, can you trust me? Why should you? I consult regularly for the pharmaceutical industry. I have on two separate occasions done a small piece of work for Bristol-Myers Squibb (unrelated to breast implants) and they are one of the manufacturers of breast implants. It is clear that I am a completely unreliable guide in this story. Instead you should trust the millionaire shysters whose only motive is philanthropic concern for breast-implant victims and whose grasp of science is so sure that they do not need data to come to their conclusions.

Case dismissed

> I am also the judge. Now would you like a long or a short sentence?'
> A short one if you please,' said Milo
> 'Good,' said the judge, rapping his gavel three times. 'I always have trouble remembering the long ones. How about 'I am'? That's the shortest sentence I know.
>
> Norton Juster The Phantom Tollbooth

But now we must move on. We have heard the cases, we have had the cross-examinations and our ten chapters are over. We call on Chapter 11 to sum up the case for statistics for the gentlemen and ladies of the jury.

11

The empire of the sum

It is not that figures lie, but that liars sometimes figure.

Maurice Kendall

Squaring up

So how has he done our 'square'? Have I persuaded you that there is more to his work than simply copying figures and pasting them into a book?[1] Are you convinced that the calculation of chances and consequences and the comprehension of contingencies are crucial to science and indeed all rational human activity? Do you now know that the figure who figures, who does all this, is the statistician?

Perhaps I have overstated the case. Statistical reasoning is a vital part of scientific activity, of that I am convinced, but statistics is no closed shop. If it is much more than simply counting and averaging, that does not mean that only statisticians are capable of doing it. In fact many with labels other than 'statistician' are busy with probability and data. Later in this chapter we shall consider some examples but first I am going to take my last chance to show you how important statistics is, whoever does it. We shall consider a recent controversy to show exactly how many of the topics we have covered in this book would be needed to resolve it.

Spots of bother

In the spring of 2002, the MMR (measles, mumps, rubella) vaccine was continuing to make headlines in the United Kingdom. The UK government was frantically trying to convince parents of the safety of this vaccine against a background of claims that the MMR vaccine placed children at risk of autism and inflammatory bowel disease. In February the Prime Minister, Tony Blair, issued a statement supporting the use of the vaccine but continued to refuse to reveal whether his own son, Leo, had been vaccinated.[2] Meanwhile, half a world away and almost entirely unnoticed in Britain,[3] an outbreak of measles was raging in the Western Highlands of Papua New Guinea. By the end of April more than 1200 children had been admitted to hospital and over 100 had died.

It was in New Guinea, nearly 60 years earlier, that the Australian Oliver Lancaster (1913–2001), then a pathologist on active wartime service, was preparing himself for a change of career.[4] He spent his evenings studying by the light of a kerosene lamp for an external course in mathematics at the University of Sydney, where he had graduated in medicine in 1937. When his war service was over, it was as an epidemiologist rather than a pathologist that he returned to civilian employment with the University of Sydney. Later, a Rockefeller fellowship enabled him to undertake a period of study at the London School of Hygiene and Tropical Medicine under Bradford Hill. Back in Australia, he realised that internal university politics would make it unlikely that he would be given a Chair in medical statistics and so he undertook further study in mathematics to qualify himself for a Chair in mathematical statistics, which he took up in 1959. Amongst his many contributions to mathematical statistics are work on the logic of significance tests and an extension of 'Cochran's Theorem' that we noted in Chapter 8. Lancaster is thus a particularly fine example of a scientific type that has featured frequently throughout this book ever since we met Daniel Bernoulli: the medic driven to mathematics.

Germane to 'German' germs

In 1941 the Sidney eye specialist, Sir Norman Gregg (1892–1968), became alarmed at the number of babies he was examining who had congenital cataracts. He overheard two of the mothers discussing that they had both had German measles in early pregnancy. Enquiries then established that of 78 children born with cataracts in the early months of 1941, 68 had been born to mothers who had had German measles in pregnancy. Gregg became convinced of a link but had difficulty in persuading the medical profession and this general scepticism was not entirely overcome until Lancaster analysed the data.[5] However, the National Health and Research Council of Australia was soon convinced that the matter required investigation and in September 1942 C. Swan, a medical researcher in South

Australia, was appointed to study the matter.[6] Letters were sent to all general practitioners in South Australia and the data revealed that there were 49 cases where a foetus had been exposed to German measles and that in 31 of these cases the baby had been born with congenital malformations. In addition to cataracts, deafness was also now recognised as a possible consequence, as was heart disease and mental retardation.

Rubella was first described by the German physician Daniel Sennert in 1619, who called it Röteln.[7] However it was not clearly distinguished from the similar but more serious, measles, until 1840 and it is really for the work of German physicians in the nineteenth century, rather than for Sennert, that rubella came to be called 'German' measles. For the hundred years from its being distinguished from measles until Gregg's work, it had never been considered to have any sequelae of consequence for either patient or foetus. It was postulated that the disease had now mutated to a more virulent form. Lancaster undertook statistical researches to investigate the phenomenon. By studying records of births of deaf children from Australia and New Zealand from the late nineteenth century onwards he was able to show that 'epidemics' of deafness were always preceded by epidemics of rubella and hence that this was a general consequence of rubella in pregnancy and not one limited to the current epidemic.[8]

Rubella is a curious disease in that unlike other common infections associated particularly with childhood such as measles, whooping cough, scarlet fever and diphtheria it very rarely has any serious *direct* consequence for child or adult. The fact that it is, nonetheless, a serious disease is precisely because of its effect on unborn children, with an extremely high risk of damage to the foetus of any woman who catches it in early pregnancy. This raises ethical issues, since the only value in immunising boys is not for any immunity granted to them, but as a contribution to the increase in 'herd immunity' in order to reduce the probability of females who have not been immunised catching rubella in pregnancy. Mumps partly restores the sacrificial parity of the sexes, since the most important consequence of this is male sterility, which sometimes follows infection in adulthood, and here it is immunisation of females that is (partly) carried out for the good of males. However, mumps carries a more serious direct threat to those infected (not just adult males) than rubella and is worth vaccinating against for that reason alone. We shall return to this issue briefly when discussing the lessons of the MMR controversy.

In his retirement Lancaster wrote two masterly books. The second, *Quantitative Methods in Biological and Medical Sciences*, deals with much of the subject matter of this one, albeit in a very different manner. The first, *Expectations of Life*,[9] is a code by code examination of the International Classification of Diseases to establish, from a historical perspective, the burden of these afflictions on mankind. We now turn to Lancaster's account of measles in that book, for it is above all measles that makes MMR a controversial topic and we need to understand a little more about the disease.

Measles tout court

I have to turn in a report every week on the number of contagious diseases I handle. Ordinarily, I handle a couple of cases of measles a week. When I report that I had eleven cases in a single day, they're liable to quarantine the whole town . . .

F. Gilbreth and E. Gilbreth Carey, *Cheaper by the Dozen*

According to Lancaster, it is generally believed that the disease of measles cannot predate, 'the development of the great agricultural and riverine civilizations'.[10] The density of population required to sustain it was not present in more primitive societies. This observation itself, of course, is dependent on the sort of understanding of the dynamics of disease, and thresholds, which requires the mathematical and statistical tools we described (very superficially) in Chapter 9.

The disease has an incubation period of 10–14 days followed by an infectious period of a few days at the onset of symptoms. Where malnutrition is common, the case fatality rate of measles can be as high as 20%. In developed countries, however, the fatality rate is low. Nevertheless, because measles is a common disease, in populations not protected by vaccination this can still translate into an important number of deaths. Figure 11.1 (which will be discussed in more detail in due course) shows deaths from measles in London for the period 1629–1939 (with some gaps) and is based on figures from Lancaster's book.[9] In 1911 there were more than 3000 deaths in London alone, a level of mortality which, were it to occur nowadays, would create a political storm. There can also be serious complications of the disease. Roughly 1 in 1000 to 2000 cases leads to measles encephalitis, the consequences of which can include severe brain damage. More common, if less serious, are ear infection and convulsions, which affect about 1 in 20 and 1 in 200 cases respectively. Two famous victims of measles were King Kamehameha II and his consort queen Kamamalu of the Sandwich Islands (Hawaii), who visited England in 1824. They were the talk of London Society in May, confined to their beds with measles in June and in their graves in July.[11]

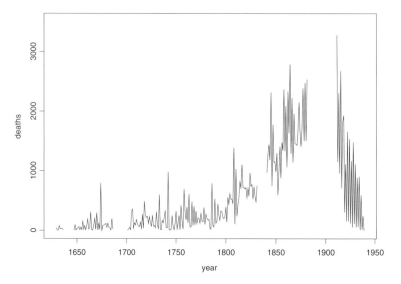

Figure 11.1 Annual deaths from measles over 300 years for London. (Based on Lancaster[9].)

What is not easily discernible from the picture presented by Figure 11.1 is the two-year cycle of the disease. This can be seen, however, by blowing up the latter part of the picture from 1911 to 1939. This has been done in Figure 11.2 to which deaths for Birmingham have also been added. A logarithmic scale has been used for deaths. The years in question are not, in fact, calendar years but are from the beginning of the preceding October to the following September and are labelled by the year in which the months January to September fall. This arrangement is convenient for isolating figures from individual epidemics and was introduced by the epidemiologist Percy Stocks (1889–1974) whose data Lancaster is quoting.[12]

The general two-year cycle is evident and initially London and Birmingham are in step, with odd years (1911, 1913, 1915) being peak years. However in London, unlike Birmingham, the epidemic of 1917 is followed immediately by another in 1918 and from then on in London it is the even years that are peak years. As might be expected with Birmingham being much smaller than London, the deaths are generally fewer. However, the peak level in Birmingham is frequently higher than the trough level in London so, because they are out of step, the lines often cross. The fact that the two peaks do not synchronise is evidence that the epidemics are largely internal to the cities concerned, with contacts between them

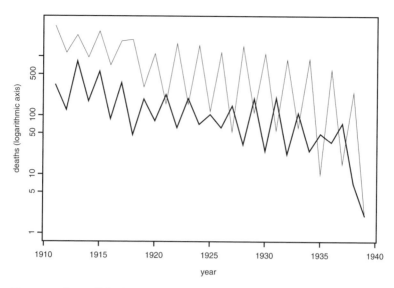

Figure 11.2 'Annual' deaths from measles in London (thin line) and Birmingham (thick line) for the period October 1910 to September 1939. Note the logarithmic axis for deaths (Based on Lancaster[13]).

being relatively unimportant. The phenomenon of the two-year cycle was extensively studied by Maurice Bartlett (1910–2002), a British mathematical statistician who followed the usual traditions of that tribe of studying at Cambridge and lecturing at University College London. In a paper of 1957 Bartlett was able to show how the pattern could arise naturally from the dynamics of the disease.[14]

To complete the trio

She held one hand to her jaw, and spoke in a dreadful whisper: 'Mumps!'

Arthur Ransome, *Winter Holiday*

Mumps has been recognised as a disease since classical times and was described by Hippocrates in the fifth century BC. It was identified as an infectious disease in the nineteenth century and in 1934 Johnson and Goodpasture were able to demonstrate that a virus in human saliva could transmit the disease to rhesus monkeys. The first safe vaccine became available in 1967.

The public health consequences of mumps are not as serious as those of either measles or rubella. It does not carry the threat of the latter to the unborn, nor that of the former to the already born, although it does threaten the 'could be born', since in adult males who catch it orchitis (inflammation of the testis) is common and this occasionally leads to sterility. Nevertheless, mumps is unpleasant, inconvenient and occasionally dangerous. Thus, given a safe vaccine it is worth immunising against. Prior to widespread immunisation mumps resulted in up to 1200 hospital admissions per year in England and Wales and in the USA was the leading identified cause of viral encephalitis. Since immunisation was introduced these problems have reduced dramatically. In recent years, however, as we have seen, the safety of the vaccine has been questioned. The MMR vaccine, which is the means by which immunity is delivered, has been attacked by patient groups and others, although, in fact, it is the measles element of this triple vaccine that is suspected by the critics of being the origin of the problem. We now look at the MMR story.

Hyperborean hyperbole?[15]

... that final land,
Where down the sky's large whitenesses, the archipelagoes of day
Gradually move, on forests light with birch and black with larch
In grave progressions ...

James Kirkup, For the 90th Birthday of Sibelius

In the 1970s epidemics of measles, mumps and rubella were common in Finland. The mean annual incidence being respectively about 350, 250 and 100 per 100 000 respectively.[16] Finland has a population of about five million and this translates into about 18 000, 12 000 and 5000 cases per year. There were hundreds of hospitalisations, an average of about 100 cases of encephalitis per year, meningitis, orchitis and sometimes sterility, especially amongst army recruits, and 40–50 annual cases of congenital birth defects due to rubella.

In 1975 a live-virus measles vaccine was introduced but since only 70% of the population was targeted, the disease was not eradicated. Military personnel had been immunised against mumps since 1960 but this was not extended to the general population. In 1982 the combined measles, mumps rubella vaccine we now know as MMR was approved in Finland.[17] It had already been used for nearly a decade in the USA. The Finns, however, embarked on a more radical and thorough programme of eradication. Children were to be vaccinated twice, aged 14–18 months and again at six years of age. The programme was accompanied by very careful data collection and study: all suspected cases of disease were tested serologically, every vaccinated person was identified by social security number, unvac-cinated children were identified by record linkage, the incidence of the three diseases was monitored carefully and a double-blind controlled trial of 1162 twins was carried out to look for side-effects.

The target population was 563 000 children. However, by 1986 only 86s% had been vaccinated. A vigorous follow-up campaign was initiated, including personal contact by public health nurses and personal letters if that failed. As a consequence a further 62 00 children were vaccinated and in total 97% received the vaccine.

The incidence of measles dropped dramatically. Such temporal coinci-dences are far from conclusive evidence of causation. Other facts support the efficacy of the programme. There was an outbreak of measles in 1988–1989, probably of foreign origin, with 1748 confirmed cases. There was a dramatic difference in incidence between vaccinated and unvaccinated age groups. Children under one year of age, who would be too young to have been vaccinated, and those aged 13 and over, who were too old for the scheme when it was introduced showed much higher rates of attack than those aged 2–12, who were in the protected cohorts. Similar evidence could be brought for the pattern of mumps and rubella infections.

The twin study showed that with the exception of transient generally mild reactions there were no detectable side-effects of the vaccine. The in-cidence of respiratory symptoms was virtually identical amongst the vac-cinated and unvaccinated. Such a study, however, would be insufficiently large to detect rare (but possibly serious) side-effects. However, follow-up of the 1.5 million Finns vaccinated from 1982 to 1993 did not turn up any problems with the vaccine. It seems that Finland had achieved a mighty victory, at relatively little cost, against three formidable foes. Other coun-tries now prepared themselves to repeat this success, amongst them, the UK.

UK OK?[18]

In 1985 the target was set in the UK eradicating indigenous measles by the year 2000. Vaccination for measles had been introduced in 1968 and rubella followed two years later. The MMR vaccine was introduced in 1988. In 1996 the Finnish policy of using a second immunisation was intro-duced. The need for a second immunisation is, ironically, due to the pro-tection which mothers are able to pass on to their children. Most moth-ers have been exposed to measles (or, if born since 1968, to a vaccine). This means that they have circulating antibodies, which are passed on to their children. These protect the children for 3–12 months and perhaps beyond in some cases. They also, however, prevent effective immunisation. This means that in a single immunisation policy you are on the horns of a dilemma. If you immunise early, the immunisation will fail in a substantial percentage of children. If you immunise late, you will leave unprotected a substantial percentage of children during a time window in which they are particularly vulnerable.[19] One solution is to immunise everybody twice: once early and once much later. An alternative would be to test children for antibodies prior to the second immunisation and only vaccinate those who were negative but this has the disadvantage of actually increasing the average number of contacts with the health service that are needed, since all children must be seen twice anyway and some three times.

The recommended schedule in the UK was to be an initial vaccination aged 12–15 months with a follow-up between ages three and five. Good progress was made in instituting this programme and in addition to targeting the new cohorts of infants a catch-up programme was begun for older children. However, in 1998, a paper appeared in *The Lancet* which, whilst it was to have minimal impact on the opinions of physicians and epidemiologists, was to prove a big hit with the Press, becoming the subject of numerous articles, television programmes and even a special publication by the satirical magazine *Private Eye*.

February, fame and infamy

But February made me shiver
with every paper I'd deliver

American Pie, Don McLean

On 28 February 1998 a paper in *The Lancet* with 13 authors, led by Dr Andrew Wakefield, reported a study on 12 children. The paper carefully described some very thorough examinations that had been carried out on these 11 boys and 1 girl, aged 3–10 who had been referred to the paediatric gastroenterology unit at the Royal Free Hospital and School of Medicine in London. Histories were taken, neurological and psychiatric assessments were made, stool and urine samples were taken, lumbar puncture, ileocolonoscopy, cerebral magnetic-resonance imaging and electroencephalography were performed.

The paper presented a number of findings, which boil down to this. First all 12 children[20] had gastrointestinal disease and developmental regression. Second in 8 of these 12 children the parents associated the onset with the child having been given MMR. There are thus two issues that the Wakefield et al. paper appears to raise. First, is gastrointestinal disease associated with developmental regression? Second, is MMR a possible cause of them both?

Now, if we think back to Sir Norman Gregg's identification of rubella in pregnancy as a cause of congenital malformations, at first sight the MMR case seems very similar. First, viruses are implicated. (MMR uses attenuated live viruses.) Second, a wide range of sequelae seem to be involved. Third, there had been a recent increase in the condition in question. Fourth, the story starts with an observational association. Surely, Wakefield et al. have stumbled on something important? Is it not hypocritical to praise Gregg and damn Wakefield?

However, closer examination shows some rather important differences between these two stories. First, the rise in the number of cataracts being seen by Gregg was much more dramatic than any recent increases in autism that Britain had experienced. Second, rubella in pregnancy is a relatively rare condition. In the period in question MMR was not at all an unusual thing for children to have been given. Wakefield's subjects must have been born between 1987 and 1995. But according to World Health Organisation figures rates of measles immunisation for the birth cohorts from 1987 ranged from 76% to 92% so that finding 12 children with autism who have received MMR is unremarkable. To put it another way, if none of the children had received MMR this would (accepting the other weaknesses of this form of study) be an indication that MMR had a protective effect against autism.

So how could the Wakefield et al. observations be explained? Very easily, as the following analogous example shows. Suppose that as a physician I develop the following hypothesis. I make it known that I believe there is a syndrome in which difficulties in breathing are associated with athlete's foot. In the course of time, due to my reputation as an expert in this area, a number of persons present at my clinic who have itchy feet and complain of shortness of breath (let us call this *chest and foot syndrome*). These individuals are examined further and spirometry reveals that their forced expiratory volume in one second is below that predicted for their height, sex and age whereas laboratory examinations confirm that the itchy red patches between their toes are tinea pedis. When asked, it turns out that most of them watch television. I then consider whether it is not possible that watching television is a cause of chest and foot syndrome.

Courting controversy

More than four years after the Wakefield paper the MMR story was still making news. *The Times* of 10 July 2002 described one of the more curious developments. Two mothers were being taken to court by the fathers of their children because they were refusing to vaccinate the children. *The Times* had campaigned for the case to be held in public as the arguments would be in the public interest. However, Mr. Justice Sumner ruled that the case should be heard in private.

What issues were considered relevant by Mr. Justice Sumner in coming to his decision?[21] Well not many, I suspect, will have to do with science and perhaps this is reasonable. Many of us, surely, will have some sympathy with the point of view that parents can decide, within limits, what is best for their children even if that decision is irrational. The problem here is that the parents don't agree. Suppose for the moment, however, that the safety or otherwise of MMR was relevant to his decision. What does the evidence show?

Since February 1998 a number of scientists have sought to test for a causal link between MMR and autism. For example, in June 1999, *The Lancet* reported an investigation[22] with a principal author from the same medical school at which Wakefield and colleagues worked: the Royal Free and University College London School, which coincidentally happens to be the one in which I have an appointment. This time, however, a serious attempt was made to examine causality and the co-authors included Paddy Farrington, a well-known statistician based at the Open University specialising in the model of infectious diseases and who had only a few years earlier published details of a statistical approach to assessing the safety or otherwise of vaccines.[23] The authors identified children with autism born since 1979 from a special needs register of eight districts of North Thames. For these children they obtained data on date of diagnosis and date of first parental concern about autism as well as immunisation records. They were able to confirm 214 cases of core autism amongst this group of children.

Taylor et al. examined their data in three different ways. First, they used the technique of Poisson regression to which we alluded in the last chapter to see whether there was a step up in the rate of development of autism for birth cohorts starting from 1987. Second, they compared age at diagnosis of autism with vaccinated and unvaccinated children to see whether there was any difference. Third, using the technique proposed by

Farrington, they looked for a possible temporal association between vaccination and the onset of autism. (The latter was measured in three different ways: dates of first *parental* concern, of medical diagnosis or of developmental regression.) For none of these approaches did they find any suggestion that MMR caused autism.

None of this has made the slightest difference to the general public who can rely on experts such as the journalists at the satirical magazine *Private Eye* to assure them that Dr. Wakefield and colleagues have proved that MMR causes autism. The fact that these very same techniques could be used to prove that reading *Private Eye* causes senility and impotence does not disturb them.

Does this mean that we know that MMR does not cause autism? No. We are faced again with the problem of Hermione. Proving something is safe is almost impossible. Conclusions of safety are always tentative and hostage to being overturned by further study. This shows the superiority of 'holistic' and 'alternative' medicine over the scientific sort. In addition to the regular emails I receive inviting me to collaborate in shifting funds from West Africa, to visit some young lady's website, to make thousands of dollars working from home, invest in some stock that is sure to go up, or increase the size of my penis or breasts, I often get offered natural Viagra. (The persons making these offers must assume that I spend my time reading *Private Eye* and am suffering from senility and impotence in consequence.) Natural Viagra has the advantage over the unnatural sort, apparently, of being perfectly safe. Why? Well because 'natural' *means* 'safe'. If ever there was a word that has become the money of fools, *natural* is it. On the same basis all female sprinters have loose sexual morals since they are all fast women. Hemlock, nightshade and tobacco are all natural and ancient remedies. (They all appear in Culpepper's *Complete Herbal and English Physician* for example.) So you can take as much as you like without harm, only don't sue me if you come to grief. I offer the following simple and consistent explanation for the persistent irrational belief that natural remedies are safe: taking them rots your brain, gradually destroying the capacity for logical thought.

Work for the diceman

Thinking more positively about the story, what does it teach us about the role of statistics in determining a rational policy for protecting populations from these diseases? What work falls to our 'square', our diceman?

First it tells us of the value of data and systems for collecting them. This is a theme that has been neglected in this work, partly because this activity is less exciting than working with probability and partly because it was the activity least in need of explanation. If there was one thing that the general public knew about statisticians it was that they collected statistics. But if the theme was not addressed it was not suppressed. It has never been far from our story. Arbuthnot could not have carried out his significance test without the data collected by the parish clerks and that particular story can be traced back to Thomas Cromwell's statistical *diktat*. Without Kaspar Neumann's compilation of data from Breslau, Halley could not have constructed his life-table. Galton's analysis of the efficacy of prayer depended on Guy's data and Pearson's meta-analysis on Simpson's. The data on measles that we have quoted from Lancaster were compiled by Stocks and Guy and, again, their collection is due to systems that owe their origins to Thomas Cromwell.

Collecting good and reliable statistics on health can be a challenging task and the science has been fortunate that from time to time scientists have been found to rise to it. For example, William Farr (1807–1883), who worked at the British General Registry Office from 1837–1880 and was a man endowed with very modest mathematical talents, registered a vital contribution to the history of vital registration. The developments he made to the collection, dissemination and interpretation of statistics were essential to the rapid progress in public health in the second half of the nineteenth century and beyond. It was Farr who convinced Florence Nightingale (1820–1910), herself an important collector of vital statistics, of the role that hospitals played in spreading disease.[24]

Turning specifically to the collection of statistics for infectious diseases there are many matters that can tax the wits of statisticians. What impact does under-reporting have on interpreting figures? What can be done to improve rates of reporting? What is the value of confirming cases by testing for seropositivity? Should we carry out surveys of seropositivity? If so, how should they be organised? How many individuals should be sampled? How frequently should samples be taken? How should they be drawn, that is to say how should the individuals to be tested be chosen?

A second task is that of statistical modelling. As we hinted in Chapter 9, but were not able to demonstrate fully, the field is so complex that good quantitative prediction is difficult at best and impossible at worst. Nevertheless qualitative but useful results may be possible. It may be feasible to give some indication as to what level of immunisation is needed for eradication. Policy as regards the necessity and timing of follow-up second immunisation can be guided by such models. As Anderson and May put it, "A central question in such programmes is what is the best age at which to vaccinate children so as to protect as many susceptibles as possible while minimizing the number of vaccinations that are 'wasted' on children who still possess significant titres of maternally derived antibodies specific to measles virus antigens".[25]

Then there is the investigation of causality, the ability to affect health for both good and harm. The statistician's standard instruments here are the clinical trial, the cohort study and the case–control study. The first of these is the design of choice for illustrating the efficacy of vaccines. An early example of its use was the American trial to test the efficacy of the Salk polio vaccine, which was reported in 1955. The biostatistician on the advisory committee of the National Foundation for Infantile Paralysis (NFIP) was none other than William G. Cochran.[26] The leaders of the NFIP wanted a non-randomised study whereby second-grade children would be offered the vaccine, and first and third year children would act as the controls. Others, including Dr. Thomas Francis a virologist and epidemiologist who had been appointed to lead the study, wanted a randomised design. At a key meeting on 11 January 1954 scientists planning the trial, after a general discussion in the morning, divided into three groups for the afternoon.[27] The clinicians reported back that they favoured observed controls, the statisticians that they favoured a placebo-controlled design. The third group, that of health officers, had been joined by Francis himself and gave support to the placebo-controlled approach. However, in the end, only eight states would support this. Eventually a compromise trial proceeded. A total of over 400 000 children were randomised to either vaccine or saline solution. More than one million further children were enrolled into the observed control study. This involved not only centres in the USA but in Canada and Finland as well.[28]

The final results of the study were as given in Table 11.1.[29]

The trial had to be huge in order to be able to prove the efficacy of the treatment and this is a general feature of clinical trials of vaccines. These suffer not only from the problem that they are trying to prevent relatively rare events from occurring, a feature that drives sample size up dramatically, but that through a contribution to herd immunity from the treated group the control group may benefit from vaccination also. When one is looking for rare and unknown side-effects, however, this prospective form of design has many difficulties. More promising is the case–control study.

Table 11.1. *Salk Polio vaccine trial (based on Bland).*

Study group	Paralytic cases	Number in group	Rate
Randomised			
Vaccine	33	200 745	16
Placebo	115	201 229	57
Refused	121	338 778	36
Observed			
Vaccine	38	221 998	17
Control	330	725 173	46
Refused	43	123 605	35

Once a suspicion has arisen of a particular side-effect, cases suffering from it are sampled and compared to controls who are not so-afflicted. The 'outcome' then in each group is the proportion of cases or controls who received the vaccine. Such studies require very careful design and analysis and provide further work for the diceman.

Then there is the question of the Law. Suppose that it were generally accepted (despite all current evidence) that MMR 'caused' autism: that is to say that children who were vaccinated had an increased risk of autism. It still would not follow that any child with autism subsequent on MMR vaccination had it caused by the vaccination. Does statistics have anything to say about this? It turns out that it does. A related task is generally carried out in the field of 'pharmacovigilence' where epidemiologists have to assess whether given adverse reactions are caused by a drug or not. This is known as 'single-case assessment' and has been studied by statisticians. For example, Tim Hutchinson, together with my colleague Phil Dawid (whose work on the Island Problem we considered in the last chapter), as well as the well-known medical statistician David Spiegelhalter and others have developed a Bayesian approach to assessing causality in such cases.[30]

Finally, through its sub-science of decision analysis, statistics has much to say about ethical and economic aspects of vaccination. Take the case being considered by Justice Sumner. One of the mothers concerned was quoted by the *Daily Mail* as saying, 'I think the safest thing for my child is to be unvaccinated in a society of vaccinated children,' to which she added, 'I'm aware this may seem selfish but this is what is in the best interests of my child and not Society at large'.[31] This is all very logical. The problem is analogous to what the ecologist Garret Hardin called 'The Tragedy of the Commons'.[32] The value to a given herdsman[33] of grazing one new animal on the common is less than the loss through the detrimental effect on all other animals. But this detriment is only relevant to his decision for those animals he owns, and if this is a small fraction of the totality of animals, he may decide to graze, against the general interest. The sum of such individual decisions produces famine. Similarly, for infectious diseases in humans, provided high levels of vaccination are maintained, it may be rational not to vaccinate one's child, even if the vaccine is probably safe because there will always be a small risk it is not.

These two cases are examples of what are referred to as *externalities* by economists: costs or benefits or both accrue to others than those taking the decisions that induce them. Under such circumstances political intervention may be necessary to ensure good decision-making. In the context of vaccination we need to know what is a rational policy? How should we encourage parents to co-operate in an era in which physicians are less trusted – mistrust of physicians being an attitude of which statisticians are far from innocent and can hardly condemn in others? This was not a problem in the era of the Salk trial, or at least it was not a general problem. Would it be logical to offer health-insurance advantages to those who agreed to vaccinate their children? What would be a fair increase in cover? Might one agree to compensate for disabilities on a no-fault basis for those who vaccinated? What arguments can one bring or arrangements can one make to encourage parents whose only children are boys to have rubella immunisation? Such a boy is not directly at risk through rubella and his unborn children are only at increased risk if the woman who conceives them is not vaccinated herself and he contributes to her infection. These are a lot of contingencies to bear in mind when making a decision.

No closed shop

Good heavens! For more than forty years I have been speaking prose without knowing it!

Moliere, *Le Bourgeois Gentilhomme*

Of course, such quantitative decision-making is not the sole preserve of statisticians. It would be foolish for any person who has the label 'statistician' to assume either that the label makes him or her a member of some calculating elite or that membership of such an elite is restricted to those with the label. However, to the extent that such decision-making does involve both the assessment of probabilities and the calculation of their consequences, any scientist who wishes to contribute, by whatever name, must think like a statistician.

There are many who think this way who do not own the label. If we go back to the generation of statisticians who graduated before the 1970s, almost none had statistics as a first degree. Before the Second World War all who made their way into the subject came via other subjects, usually, but not exclusively, mathematics. Neyman and the two Pearsons were mathematicians. de Finetti was a mathematician with an interest in economics and genetics.[34] Fisher was a mathematician but it was really his interest in genetics and evolution that provided much of the impetus for his work in statistics and he made important contributions in these fields of biology. Student studied mathematics and chemistry at Oxford but it was really the latter that qualified him to work for Guinness, where problems of sampling led to his interest in statistics. Jeffreys was an astronomer and geophysicist whose interest in statistics can partly be traced to the courses in philosophy that he took while an undergraduate in Cambridge and also to practical problems of measurement in his scientific work.

If we need evidence that statistics is no closed shop we need look no further than the modelling of infectious diseases. The work probably best known to the general public was carried out by the biologist Roy Anderson and the physicist Robert May.[19] But there is still a debt owed to statistics. Anderson worked with the statistician Bartlett, a pioneer in the field of modelling of disease, and the influential text of Anderson and May we have already cited has plenty of references to important work by Bailey, Barbour, Becker, Cox and Dietz, all of whom could be called statisticians in the widest application of the word.

Economists have also made important contributions to statistics and statisticians have not always recognised this properly. Ramsey's pioneering Bayesian work was presented as a contribution to economics and as a reply to Keynes. Savage's work on utility was strongly influenced by economists, Chicago having a particularly strong school in the subject. I predict that impressive financial mathematics on the pricing of financial derivatives, which has its origins in the work of Fischer Black, and Nobel Prize winners Myron Scholes and Robert Merton,[35] will in turn have an important influence on the work of statisticians involved in medical decision-making. Recently Glen Shafer and Vladimir Vovk wrote a book that re-axiomises probability in terms of game theory and applies this in turn to finance.[36] What profession do the authors belong to? It is difficult to say and really doesn't matter. Shafer could be described as a statistician but also perhaps as a philosopher. 'Mathematician' might be the best description for Vovk but he works in a computing department and could also be described as a statistician. However, their work is partly inspired by that of my colleague Phil Dawid in developing the *prequential principle* and Dawid is Pearson Professor of Statistics at University College. (The prequential principle is the deceptively simple but consequential and fruitful notion that forecasting systems should only be judged by their success or otherwise in forecasting.)

Vovk is not the only person in a computing department working on probabilistic and statistical problems. Many computer scientists working in the field of artificial intelligence and machine-learning have been developing, and sometimes re-discovering, Bayesian methods. Here again there is much that statisticians could learn. In defence of my profession, however, the traffic is not all one way. Data-mining and bioinformatics have also been mainly developed by computer scientists but it might be claimed that here the cow is on the other alp and computer scientists could learn by studying statistics. A cynical definition of bioinformatics is *a synergistic fusion of huge data-bases and bad statistics* and for data-mining is *panning for gold in a sewer* and some of the hype associated with these fields, if nothing else, will not stand up to cynical statistical examination. Nevertheless, if some such work could be done better if use were made of existing statistical theory, much useful work is being done and some of it concerns matters that statisticians were initially too fastidious to tackle.

The lore of large numbers

In short, with methodical data collection, the building of huge data-bases, the increasing care and attention being paid to carrying out statistical investigations, international co-operation via organisations such as the Cochrane and Campbell Collaborations, the increase in computing power, the further development of statistical theory and algorithms and their implementation in statistical packages, we are at the birth of a golden age for statistics.

Endgame

. . . the man of the future is the man of statistics and the master of economics . . .
Oliver Wendel Holmes Jr.[37]

As the great statistician David Cox has pointed out, a golden stage for statistics is not necessarily a golden age for statisticians.[38] In a sense, it doesn't matter. Fashions come and go. We no longer call a pharmacist an apothecary but medicines are still dispensed by individuals who are required to understand their properties. 'A rose by any other name would smell as sweet', but pharmacist or apothecary, camphor has the same pungency.

An understanding of data and statistical inference, the ability to design critical experiments or collect relevant samples, a cool head and a certain cynical detachment are all necessary for good decision-making in the face of uncertainty. These are what the statistician has to offer. Dicing with death is a difficult game we have no choice but to play. The individuals who have so far paid most attention to its rules are called statisticians. Maybe others will make the moves in the future. However, it is the contribution of those who have played the game most seriously so far that we have honoured in this book.

Notes

Notes to Chapter 1

1. ICH E6 (1996) *Guideline for Good Clinical Practice*.
2. Wallace, W. A. Fortnightly review: managing in flight emergencies. *British Medical Journal* 1995; **311**: 374–375 (5 August).
3. Rogers, J. L. and Doughty, D. Does having boys or girls run in the family? *Chance* 2001; **14**: 8–13.
4. The probability given here is an exact calculation based on the binomial distribution.
5. However, the essence of Bayesian approaches to statistics is that they permit updating of belief in the light of evidence. In such a sequence of trials, for all but the most obstinately prejudiced, the probability would change.
6. See, for example, Feinstein, A. R., Sosin, D. A. and Wells, C. K. The Will Rogers phenomenon: improved technologic diagnosis and stage migration as a source of nontherapeutic improvement in cancer prognosis. *Transactions of the Association of American Physicians* 1984; **97**: 19–24.
7. This section benefits considerably from an excellent paper by Milo Schield: Schield, M. Simpson's paradox and Cornfield's conditions. *ASA-JSM* 1999. http://www.Statlit.org/Articles.htm.
8. The interpretation of interactions in contingency tables. *Journal of the Royal Statistical Society B* 1951; **13**: 238–241.
9. Pearson, K., Lee, A. and Bramley-Moore, L. Genetic (reproductive) selection: inheritance of fertility in man. *Philosophical Transactions of the Royal Society A* 1899; **73**: 534–539.
10. Julious, S. A. and Mullee, M. A. Confounding and Simpson's paradox. *British Medical Journal* 1994; **309**: 1480–1481.
11. Pearl, J. *Causality*. Cambridge University Press, 2000.
12. Alan Dershowitz, as quoted by Garfield, J. B. and Snell, J. L. *Journal of Statistics Education* v.3, n.2 (1995). See http://www.stat.unipg.it/ncsu/info/jse/v3n2/resource.html.
13. Good, I. J. When batterer turns murderer. *Nature* 1995; **375**: 541.
14. Merz, J. F. and Caulkins, J. P. Propensity to abuse – propensity to murder? *Chance* 1995; **8**: 14.

15. A song with this title sung by Crystal Gayle got to number 5 in the British single charts in 1977.

16. Cochrane, A. L. *Effectiveness and Efficiency. Random Reflections on Health Services.* Postcript, The Royal Society of Medicine Press, 1971.

Notes to Chapter 2

1. Of course, by *numbers* Pope means verses.

2. His name is sometimes spelled Arbuthnott.

3. Shoesmith, E. In Johnson, N. L. and Kotz, S. *Leading Personalities in Statistical Sciences.* Wiley, 1997.

4. *Philosophical Transactions* 1710; **27**: 186–90. As Hacking, *The Emergence of Probability*, Cambridge, 1975 points out (p. 167), Arbuthnot's data include births up to the end of 1710, so that the official publication date of 1710 must be too early.

5. This variation probably reflects differences in religious fashions over the period. Many Protestant sects did not practise infant baptism.

6. Based on Table 2.2 of Haigh, J. *Taking Chances: Winning with Probability.* Oxford University Press, 1999.

7. To calculate this we take a binomial distribution, with $n = 219$ trials, $p = 0.516$ probability of success and calculate the probability that x, the number of successes, will be less than or equal to 109. This probability is 0.318.

8. Bernoulli numbers are the coefficients of the terms defined by a particular power series.

9. Stigler, S. *The History of Statistics. The Measurement of Uncertainty before 1900.* Belknap, 1986.

10. Boyer, C. B. *A History of Mathematics* (second edition revised by Merzbach, U. C.). Wiley, 1989.

11. Bell, E. T. *Men of Mathematics.* Penguin, 1953.

12. We should not, of course, forget Frau Bernoulli's role in this. It may be that the mathematical genes or environment are all down to her.

13. Irigaray, L. *Ce Sexe Qui n'en Est Pas Un.* Editions de Minuit, 1977.

14. Sokal, A. and Bricmont, J. *Impostores Intellectuelles.* Editions Odile Jacob, 1997, pp. 159–167.

15. Bell (see note 11).

16. Source: Mathcad table of constants.

17. Sheynin, O. D. Bernoulli's work on probability. *RETE* 1972; **1**: 274–275.

18. Bernoulli, D. Sur le probleme propose pour la seconde fois par l'Acadamie Royale des Sciences de Paris. In Speiser, D. (ed.) *Die Werke von Daniel Bernoulli*, Band 3. Birkhäuser Verlag, 1987.

19. This latter feature, involving as it does the probability of events that did not occur, has made the significance tests particularly objectionable to Bayesians.

20. Trader, R. L. In Johnson and Kotz pp. 11–14, says London (see note 3). Holland, J. D. The Reverend Thomas Bayes, F. R. S. (1702–1761). *Journal of the Royal Statistical Society A* 1962; **125**: 451–461, says Hertfordshire.

21. Dale, A. I. *A History of Inverse Probability.* Springer, 1991, p. 3.

22. Trader, R. L. (See notes 3 & 20).

23. RA Fisher to E. T. Williams 31 October 1953. See Bennett, J. H. (ed.) *Statistical Inference and Analysis. Selected Correspondence of RA Fisher.* Oxford, University Press, 1990, p. 8.

24. The Valencia of the Valencia conferences has a virtual rather than geographical reality. The 2002 meeting was held in The Canary Islands.
25. Johnson and Kotz pp. 255–256 (see note 3).
26. Among Greek symbols, θ is a fairly popular choice for a probability.
27. *Alices Adventures in Wonderland*, chapter 7.
28. The Laplace transform is a particular mathematical device used in the solution of differential equations.
29. Gillespie, C. C. *Pierre-Simon Laplace, 1749–1827. A Life in Exact Science*. Princeton University Press, 1997.
30. *Sartor Resartus*, 1838. Although mainly known as a literary figure Carlyle was also a mathematician and translated the *Eléments de Géométrie* of Adrian Legendre (1752–1833) into English.
31. Boyer, C. B. *A History of Mathematics*, 2nd edition. Wiley, 1991.
32. Bell (see note 11).
33. Grattan-Guinness, I. In Johnson and Kotz, pp. 49–54 (see note 3).
34. Quoted in Dale p. 148. Translated Senn (see note 21).
35. Quoted in Dale p. 166. Translated Senn (see note 21).
36. Arthur Barker Limited, London, 1963.
37. Box, J. F. *RA Fisher, The Life of a Scientist*. Wiley, 1978, p. 8.
38. Ibid, p. 17.
39. Ibid, p. 33.
40. Dawkins, R. *The Blind Watchmaker*. Penguin, 1988, p. 199.
41. David, F. N. In Johnson and Kotz, pp. 150–152 (see note 3).
42. Scott, E. In Johnson and Kotz, pp. 137–145 (see note 3).
43. *Biometrika* 1908; 6: 1–25.
44. Pearson, E. S. *Student. A Statistical Biography of William Sealy Gosset*. Clarendon Press, 1990.
45. Senn, S. J. and Richardson, W. The first *t*-test. *Statistics in Medicine* 1994; **13**: 783–803.
46. Fisher, R. A. *Statistical Methods for Research Workers*. Oliver and Boyd, 1925.
47. Lindley, D. V. In Johnson and Kotz, pp. 128–129 (see note 3).
48. See, for example, Pearson, K. On the criterion that a given system of deviations from the probable in the case of a correlated system of variables is such that it can be reasonably supposed to have arisen from random sampling. *Philosophical Magazine* 1900; **50**: 157–175.

Notes to Chapter 3

1. Armitage, P. Obituary: Sir Austin Bradford Hill, 1897–1991. *Journal of the Royal Statistical Society A* 1991; **154**: 482–484.
2. A. V. Hill, a UCL man, is famous to all pharmacologists as the originator of the Hill equation much-used in modelling the dose–response of pharmaceuticals.
3. Whom we shall encounter in Chapter 9.
4. Johnson, N. L. and Kotz, S. *Leading Personalities in Statistical Sciences*. Wiley, 1997.
5. Johnson and Kotz, p. 334.
6. Box, J. F. *RA Fisher, The Life of a Scientist*. Wiley, 1978, p. 33.
7. Box, J. F., pp. 35–37.
8. Box, J. F., p. 57 and Bennet, J. H. *Natural Selection, Heredity and Eugenics*. Clarendon Press, 1983, p. 214.
9. Box, J. F., plate 7.

10. Collected Papers 48. The arrangement of field experiments. *Journal of the Ministry of Agriculture of Great Britain* 1926; **33**: 503–513.
11. Box, J. F., pp. 131–135.
12. According to Joan Fisher Box. However, I am not convinced that the disagreement as to the preferable order of tea and milk was this way round.
13. Stigler, S. Stigler's law of eponomy. *Transactions of the New York Academy of Sciences, 2nd series* 1980; **39**: 147–157.
14. Kline, M. *Mathematical Thought from Ancient to Modern Times*, volume 1, Oxford University Press, 1972, p. 273.
15. Edwards, A. W. F. *Pascal's Arithmetical Triangle*. The Johns Hopkins University Press, 1987, 2002.
16. Edwards ibid, p. xiii.
17. Lilford, R. J. and Jackson, J. Equipoise and the ethics of randomization. *Journal of the Royal Society of Medicine* 1995; **88**: 552–559.
18. First published 1972. Oxford University Press paperback 1973.
19. Trochim, W. M. K. and Capelleri, J. C. Cutoff strategies for enhancing randomized clinical trials. *Controlled Clinical Trials* 1992; **13**: 190–212.
20. See, for example, Senn, S. J. *Statistical Issues in Drug Development*. Wiley, 1997.
21. See, for example, Berry, D. and Eick, S. Adaptive assignment versus balanced randomization in clinical trials: a decision analysis. *Statistics in Medicine* 1995; **14**: 231–246.
22. International Conference on Harmonisation, ICH Harmonised Tripartite Guideline E10, Choice of control group and related issues, 2000.

Notes to Chapter 4

1. Littlewood is referring to Bertrand Russell. See *Littlewood's Miscellany*, Cambridge University Press, 1986, p. 128.
2. Hume, D. *My own Life*. 1776, Chapter 1.
3. Quinton, A. *Hume*. Phoenix Press, 1998.
4. Hume, D. *A Treatise of Human Nature*, Book I, section XI. First published 1739 and 1740. My edition was published by Penguin in 1969.
5. Laplace, P. S. *A Philosophical Essay on Probabilities*. Translated by Truscott, F. W. and Emory, F. L. Dover, 1951, p. 19.
6. 'This feorful worm wad often feed On calves an' lambs an' sheep, An' swally little bairns alive When they laid doon to sleep.' etc. See for example the web pages of Sunderland University at http://www.sunderland.ac.uk/lambton.html.
7. Cook, A. *Sir Harold Jeffreys, Biographical Memoirs of Fellows of the Royal Society* 1990; **36**: 303–333.
8. Box, J. F. *RA Fisher, The Life of a Scientist*. Wiley, 1978, pp. 439–440.
9. In praise of Bayes. *The Economist*, September 2000.
10. Jeffreys, H. *Theory of Probability* third edition. Oxford, 1961, pp. 127–128.
11. Jeffreys, H. *ibid.*, p. 129.
12. Johnson, N. L. and Kotz, S. *Leading Personalities in Statistical Sciences*. Wiley, 1997, p. 266.
13. Ramsey, F. P. Truth and probability (1926). In Braithwaite, R. B. (ed.) *The Foundations of Mathematics and Other Logical Essays*. Kegan, Paul, Trench, Trubner and Co. Harcourt Brace, 1931, Chapter VII, pp. 156–198.

14. Savage, J. L. *The Foundations of Statistics*. Originally published by Wiley, 1954. I have used the Dover edition, Toronto 1972.

15. Smith, A. A conversation with Dennis Lindley. *Statistical Science*, 1995; **10**: 305–319.

16. Dawid, A. P., Stone, M. and Zidek, J. V. Marginalisation paradoxes in Bayesian and structural inference. *Journal of the Royal Statistical Society, B*. 1973; **35**: 189–233.

17. Lee, J. A. N. at http://ei.cs.vt.edu/~history/Good.html.

18. de Finetti, B. D. *Theory of Probability*, volume 1. Wiley, 1974. Translated by Machi, A. and Smith, A.

19. From the English translation by Di Maio, M. C., Galavotti, M. C. and Jeffrey, R. C. Probabilism. *Erkenntnis* 1989; **31**: 169–223. The quotation can be found on p. 219.

20. La prèvision: ses lois logiques, ses sources subjectives. *Annales de l'Institut Henri Poincaré* 1937; **7**: 1–68.

21. de Finetti, B. D. *Theory of Probability*, volume 1. Wiley, 1974, p. 161. Translated by Machi, A. and Smith, A.

22. Reid, C. *Neyman from Life*. Springer, 1982.

23. Scott, E. In Johnson and Kotz, pp. 137–138 (see note 12).

24. On the problem of the most efficient tests of statistical hypotheses. *Philosophical Transactions of the Royal Society, Series A* 1933; **231**: 289–337.

25. A suggestion of Tocher's. Tocher, K. D. Extension of the Neyman-Pearson theory of tests to discontinuous variates.*Biometrika* 1950; **37**: 130–144.

26. A result proved by Pitman, E. J. G. *Some Remarks on Statistical Inference: Bernoulli, Bayes, Laplace*. Springer, 1965, pp. 209–216. See also Barnard, G. *Statistics in Medicine* 1990; **9**: 601–614.

27. Popper, K. *Unended Quest*. Routledge, 1974.

28. de Finetti, B. D. *Theory of Probability*, volume 1, Wiley, 1974, p. 141. Translated by Machi, A. and Smith, A.

29. Phil Dawid, a colleague at UCL, has tried to develop such a theory. See Dawid, A. P. Probability, causality and the empirical world: a Bayes–de Finetti–Popper–Borel synthesis. *UCL Statistical Science Research Report* No. 228.

30. Barnard, G. A. Fragments of a statistical autobiography. *Student* 1996; **1**: 257–268.

Notes to Chapter 5

1. Henry, D. A., Smith, A. J. and Hennessy, S. Basic principles of clinical pharmacology relevant to pharmacoepidemiology studies. In Strom, B. L. (ed.) *Pharmacoepidemiology*. Wiley; 1995, pp. 39–56.

2. See, for example, Lilja, J. J., Kivisto, K. T. and Neuvonen, P. J. Grapefruit juice increases serum concentrations of atorvastatin and has no effect on pravastatin. *Clinical Pharmacology and Therapeutics* 1999; **66**: 118–127.

3. Hennekens, C. H. and Eberlein, K. A randomized trial of aspirin and beta-carotene among U.S. physicians. *Preventive Medicine* 1985; **14**: 165–168.

4. The National Institutes of Health Revitalization Amendments of 1992 (Senate – October 05, 1992). Available online at http://thomas.loc.gov/home/thomas.html.

5. Meinert, C. L., Gilpin, A. K., Unalp, A. and Dawson, C. Gender representation in trials. *Controlled Clinical Trials* 2000; **21**: 462–475.

6. NIH Revitalization Act of 1993, Public Law 103–43, Reprinted in Mastroianni, A. C., Faden, R. and Federman, D. (eds.) *Women and Health Research*, volume 1. National Academy Press, 1994.

7. Laplace, P. S. *A Philosophical Essay on Probabities*. Translated by Truscott, F. W. and Emory, F. L. Dover, 1951.

Notes to Chapter 6

1. This was true at the time of writing. In autumn 2003 I took up a chair at Glasgow University.
2. Your author must hang his head in shame. He was not good enough for Cambridge even before he was a statistician.
3. There are some notable exceptions to this journalistic incompetence. The famous American statistician, Harold Hotelling, originally studied journalism. Robert Matthews, the science correspondent of the *Sunday Telegraph*, has done some interesting research in approaches to interpreting statistical evidence. I do not know if Mr. Victor Lewis Smith of *The Evening Standard* has any statistical training but he seems, remarkably, to be immune to the sort of nonsense that regularly gulls his colleagues.
4. Zobel, G. *The Big Issue*. August 30–September 5, 1999, pp. 6–7.
5. *The Big Issue*. 13–19 September 1999, p. 82.
6. *A Tract on Monetary Reform*, 1923. Actually, the long run has a technical meaning to economists as being the period in which the conditions of supply can change. In terms of human life this might be one generation, in which case, in pedantic mood, one might say that in at most four or five long runs we are all dead.
7. 'Hegel says somewhere that all great events and personalities in world history reappear in one fashion or another. He forgot to add the first time as tragedy, the second as farce.' *The Eighteenth Brumaire of Louis Bonaparte*, 1852.
8. *Almost surely* does not imply here that some will nearly die but, in the parlance of the probabilist, that the probability that none will die, although not zero, is effectively zero.
9. Wilde, O. *The Importance of Being Earnest*, Act Two.
10. This section is largely indebted to Forrest's book, *The Life and Work of a Victorian Genius*, Paul Elek, 1974.
11. Forrest, ibid, p. 111.
12. This paper is available on the web thanks to Abelard at http://www.abelard.org/galton/galton.htm#prayer.
13. Brownlee, K. A. *Industrial Experimentation*. HMSO, 1946.
14. Dodge, Y. The guinea pig of multiple regression. In Rieder, H. (ed.) *Robust Statistics, Data Analysis and Computer Intensive Methods*. Springer-Verlag, pp. 91–117.
15. Fisher, R. A. Collected Papers 138. The use of multiple measurement in taxonomic problems. *Annals of Eugenics* 1936; **7**: 179–188.
16. Moran, P. A. P. The statistical analysis of the Canadian lynx cycle I. *Australian Journal of Zoology* 1953; **1**: 163–173.
17. On the duration of life as affected by the pursuits of literature, science, and art: with a summary view of the duration of life among the upper and middle classes of society. *Journal of the Statistical Society of London September* 1859; **22** (3): 337–361.
18. Obituary: Dr. William A Guy. *Journal of the Statistical Society of London* 1885; **48** (4): 650–651.
19. The data Galton quotes from Guy's paper are themselves based on an earlier paper of Guy's: On the duration of life among the English gentry, with additional

observations on the duration of life among the aristocracy. *Journal of the Statistical Society of London* 1846; **9** (1): 37–49.

20. Joyce, C. R. B. and Weldon, R. M. C. The objective efficacy of prayer: a double-blind clinical trial. *Journal of Chronic Diseases* 1965; **18**: 367–377.

21. My discussion of smoking and lung cancer is particularly indebted to the helpful discussion by Freedman, D. From association to causation: some remarks on the history of statistics. *Statistical Science* 1999; **14**: 243–258.

22. Raleigh was imprisoned for treason in 1603 on James's accession. The Counterblaste dates from 1604. Raleigh was released in 1617 for the Orinoco expedition and when this failed beheaded in 1618.

23. Doll, R. and Hill, A. B. Smoking and carcinoma of the lung. *British Medical Journal* 1950; **2**: 739.

24. Wynder, E. L. and Graham, E. A. Tobacco smoking as a possible etiologic factor in bronchogenic carcinoma. *Journal of the American Medical Association* 1950; **143**: 329–336.

25. Reprinted as Schairer, E. and Schoniger, E. Lung cancer and tobacco consumption. *International Journal of Epidemiology* 2001; **30**: 24–27.

26. Fisher, R. A. Collected papers 270 Dangers of cigarette smoking. *British Medical Journal* 1957; **2**: 297–298.

27. Atkins, W. R. B. and Fisher, R. A. *Journal of the Royal Army Medical Corps* 1943; **83**: 251–252. (Fisher Collected Papers 195.)

28. Freedman, D. From association to causation: some remarks on the history of statistics. *Statistical Science* 1999; **14** (**3**): 243–258.

29. Kaprio, J. and Kosenvuo, M. Twins, smoking and mortality: a 12 year prospective study of discordant twin pairs. *Social Science and Medicine* 1989; **29**: 1083–1089.

30. Cornfield, J., Haenszel, W., Hammond, E., Lilienfeld, A., Shimkin, M., and Wynder, E. Smoking and lung cancer: recent evidence and a discussion of some questions. Journal of the National Cancer Institute 1959; **22**: 173–203.

Notes to Chapter 7

1. However, it was not part of the original correspondence of 1654 but was posed by Pascal in a letter to Fermat of 1656. See Anthony Edwards's extremely scholarly study, *Pascal's Arithmetic Triangle*, Johns Hopkins University Press, 2002 (Originally Oxford University Press, 1987). See also Edwards, A. W. F. *International Statistical Review* 1983; **51**: 73–79.

2. See Hald, A. *A History of Probability and Statistics and their Applications before 1750*. Wiley, 1990, p. 76.

3. I am extremely grateful to Isabel Trevenna of the Office for National Statistics for having provided me with data that enabled me to reconstruct my calculations of 25 years ago.

4. This was in 1698, before her accession in 1702 . Her son the Duke of Gloucester slipped in the mud.

5. Aubrey, J. *Brief Lives*. Folio Society, 1975.

6. Newton, I. *Philosophiae Naturalis Principia Mathematica*, 1687.

7. Glaisher, 1888. Cited in the *Oxford Dictionary of National Biography*. Oxford University Press.

8. This account is largely based on that by Hald (see note 2) but also greatly aided by Ed Stephan's web pages on William Graunt: http://www.ac.wwu.edu/~stephan/Graunt/bills.html.

9. From the preface of 'Natural and Political OBSERVATIONS Mentioned in a following INDEX, and made upon the Bills of Mortality' by John Graunt. This is conveniently available at http://www.ac.wwu.edu/~stephan/Graunt/bills.html.

10. *The Oxford Companion to British History*. Oxford University Press, 1997, pp. 264–265.

11. An Estimate of the Degrees of Mortality of Mankind, drawn from curious Tables of the Births and Funerals at the City of Breslau, with an attempt to ascertain the Price of Annuities upon Lives. Available online courtesy of Mathias Boehne at http://www.pierre-marteau.com/contributions/boehne-01/halley-mortality-1.html.

12. Hald, A. (see note 2).

13. According to the *Guinness British Hit Singles* (12th edition), this single reached number 7 in the British charts in August 1981.

14. Cox, D. R. Regression models and life-tables (with discussion). *Journal of the Royal Statistical Society Series B* 1972; **34**: 187–220.

15. But Benjamin, in discussion of Cox (see note 14), points out that this is not always the case.

16. Downton, F. In discussion of Cox (see note 14).

17. http://www.gm.com/company/gmability/ philanthropy/cancer_research/ ketwin9000.htm.

Notes to Chapter 8

1. This section is based mainly on Filon's Royal Society obituary and on Florence Nightingale David's biographical note in Johnson, N. L. and Kotz, S. *Leading Personalities in Statistical Sciences*. Wiley, 1997.

2. Speeches delivered at a dinner held in University College London in honour of Professor Karl Pearson, 23 April, 1934: privately printed at the University Press, Cambridge, 1934, p. 19. Also cited by Filon.

3. Magnello, E. Karl Pearson, reprinted in Heyde and Seneta. In *Statisticians of the Centuries*. Springer-Verlag, 2001.

4. Speeches delivered at a dinner held in University College London in honour of Professor Karl Pearson, 23 April, 1934: privately printed at the University Press, Cambridge, 1934, p. 19. Also cited by Filon.

5. Speeches delivered at a dinner held in University College London in honour of Professor Karl Pearson, 23 April, 1934: privately printed at the University Press, Cambridge, 1934, p. 23.

6. Karl Pearson is, of course, a vitally important figure in the history of statistics. I am grateful to Iain Chalmers, however, to having drawn my attention to his importance for the history of meta-analysis. See also Chalmers, I., Hedges, L. V. and Cooper, H. A brief history of research synthesis. *Evaluation and the Health Professions* 2002; **25**: 12–37.

7. Report on certain enteric fever inoculation statistics provided by Lieutenant-Colonel R. J. S. Simpson, C. M. G., R. A. M. C., by Karl Pearson, F. R. S. *British Medical Journal*, November 5, 1904; pp. 1243–1246.

8. This was first introduced by Pearson in *Philosophical Transactions of the Royal Society of London, Series A* 1900; **195**: 1–47.

9. Fifty percent of the Normal distribution lies between -0.6745 and 0.6745 standard errors of the mean so that if we take the standard error and multiply it by 0.6745 we obtain the probable error.

10. This section is indebted to Gene Glass's 1999 account of the genesis of meta-analysis: 'Meta-Analysis at 25' available at http://glass.ed.asu.edu/gene/papers/meta25.html.

11. Eysenck, H. The effects of psychotherapy. *International Journal of Psychotherapy* 1965; **1**: 97–178.

12. Fisher, R. A. *Statistical Methods for Research Workers*, fourth edition. Oliver and Boyd, 1934.

13. Mantel, N. and Haenszel, W. Statistical aspects of the analysis of data from retrospective studies of diseases. *Journal of the National Cancer Institute* 1959; **22**: 719–746.

14. Yates, F. and Cochran, W. G. The analysis of groups of experiments. *The Journal of Agricultural Science* 1938; **XXVIII(IV)**: 556–580.

15. Cochran, W. G. The distribution of quadratic forms in a normal system. *Proceedings of the Cambridge Philosophical Society* 1934; **30**: 178–189.

16. Cited in Biographical Memiors, V.56, 1987, p. 68. National Academy of Sciences, http://books.nap.edu/books/0309036933/html/60.html.

17. Archie Gemmill's famous goal was made the subject of a ballet by Andy Howitt who watched it (the goal) on television as a 13-year-old with his grandfather, who then promptly died from the excitement. Cochrane speculated that intensive coronary care units were bad for patients due to the fear factor. Clearly there is a connection between these two facts!

18. This account is based on the obituary of Cochrane by 'ALC' (that is to say Cochrane himself) included in Cochrane's 1971 book *Effectiveness and Efficiency, Random Reflections on the Health Services*. The Royal Society for Medicine Press, in the 1999 edition as well as on that book itself.

19. Cochrane, A. L. *Effectiveness and Efficiency, Random Reflections on the Health Services*. The Royal Society for Medicine Press, 1999, pp. 4–6.

20. Cochrane, A. L. 1931–1971: a critical review, with particular reference to the medical profession. In *Medicines for the Year 2000*. Office of Health Economics, 1979, pp. 1–11. Quoted by Iain Chalmers is his introduction to the 1999 edition of *Effectiveness and Efficiency* (see note 19).

21. *The Cochrane Collaboration: a Brief Introduction*, at www.cochrane.org/software/docs/leaflet.rtf.

22. It may be that the true author of this *bon mot* is Maurice Chevalier rather than W. C. Fields.

23. Sackett, D. L., Richardson, W. S., Rosenberg, W. and Haynes, R. B. *Evidence Medicine: How to Practice and Teach EBM*. Churchill Livingstone, 1997.

24. Smith, A. F. M. Mad cows and ecstasy. Chance and choice in an evidence-based society. *Journal of the Royal Statistical Society, A* 1996; **159**: 367–383.

25. See www.campbell.gse.upenn.edu.

Notes to Chapter 9

1. Pascal, *Pensées*. Le nez de Cléopâtre: s'il eût été plus court, toute la face de la terre aurait changé.

2. I am grateful to the late Rev. Dr. Basil Hall, one-time dean of St. John's Cambridge, for bringing this to my attention.

3. Laplace, P. S. *A Philosophical Essay on Probabilities*. Translated by Truscott, F. W. and Emory, F. L. Dover, 1951, Chapter IX.

4. See Hald, A. *A History of Mathematical Statistics from 1750 to 1930*. Wiley, 1998, p. 193.

5. The mid point between $1/4$ and $1/3$ is $7/24$. Since $175 = 600 \times 7/24$, this marks the boundary between closer agreement in number of heads to D'Alembert's probability compared to the 'standard' result. Given the 'standard' probability of $1/4$, in 600 trials the binomial distribution indicates that one would expect two heads to occur fewer than 175 times with approximately 99% probability. However, all this presupposes that the tosses are independent and fair and I have no control of the way that the reader will toss a coin!

6. Let the probability of one head be θ so that the probability of two heads is θ^2. Every value between 0 and 1 being equally likely, we can find the definite integral between 0 and 1 of θ^2 with respect to θ, $\int_0^1 \theta^2 d\theta$. This is $1/3$.

7. This is a concept that was extensively developed by my colleague Phil Dawid in a famous paper published in 1979 (*Journal of the Royal Statistical Society, B* 1979; **41**: 1–31.)

8. From one point of view, a given sequence is a single (if composite) event.

9. DeGroot, M. H. A Conversation with Persy Diaconis. *Statistical Science* 1986; **1**: 319–334.

10. Azzalini, A., Bowman, A. W. A look at some data on the Old Faithful geyser. *Journal of the Royal Statistical Society C, Applied Statistics* 1990; **39** (3): 357–365.

11. Obituary. *Lancet* 15 October, 1949.

12. Gani, J. Three pioneers of epidemic modelling: Daniel Bernoulli (1700–1782), Pyotr Dimitrievich En'ko (1844–1916), Anderson Gray McKendrick (1876–1943). Statistics Research Report No. SRR 012–96.

13. Lancaster, H. O. *Quantititative Methods in Biological and Medical Sciences*. Springer, 1994, p. 147.

14. Greenwood, M. On the statistical measure of infectiousness. *Journal of Hygiene Cambridge* 1931; **31**: 336–351.

15. Obituary notice of the Royal Society.

16. Quoted in the Royal Society obituary.

17. From 'the Place of Mathematics in Medical and Biological Statistics', Journal of the Royal Statistical Society. A presidential address for the Royal Statistical Society by J. Oscar Irwin, Bradford Hill's successor in that position.

18. Gani, J. Three pioneers of epidemic modelling: Daniel Bernoulli (1700–1782), Pyotr Dimitrievich En'ko (1844–1916), Anderson Gray McKendrick (1876–1943), Statistics Research Report No. SRR 012–96.

19. This section is based on, Davidson, J. N. *Biographical Memoirs of Fellows of The Royal Society*, **17**, November 1971 and on appendices to that obituary by McCrea and Yates.

20. This account is indebted to that of Daley, D. J. and Gani, J. *Epidemic Modelling: an Introduction*. Cambridge University Press, 1999.

21. See http://mam2000.mathforum.org/epigone/matematica/ whixdandswou.

22. See, in particular, Lancaster, H. O. *Quantitative Methods in Biological and Medical Sciences*. Springer, 1994, chapter 12.

23. These biographical notes based on The Wheaton Archives http://www.wheaton. edu/bgc/archives/GUIDES/178.htm.

24. See, for example, Hayward, J. Mathematical modeling of church growth. *Journal of Mathematical Sociology* 1999; **23**: 255–292.

25. Mary Mallon, a cook in Oyster Bay New York who is known to have infected 53 people.

Notes to Chapter 10

1. 'It is incident to physicians, I am afraid, beyond all other men, to mistake subsequence for consequence,' according to Dr. Johnson, who also said, 'Notes are often necessary but they are necessary evils'.

2. Let A be the hypothesis *trauma causes MS* and let B be *study suggests trauma causes MS*, with B' = *study does not suggest trauma cause MS*. Then since $A = (A \cap B) \cup (A \cap B')$ and $(A \cap B)$ and $(A \cap B')$ are mutually exclusive $P(A) = P(A \cap B) + P(A \cap B')$ (eq. 1). However, $P(A \mid B) > P(A)$. Thus, by Bayes theorem $P(A \cap B)/P(B) > P(A)$ from which $P(A \cap B) > P(A)P(B)$. Substituting in (1) we have $P(A) > P(A)P(B) + P(A \cap B')$ which we write as $P(A)[1 - P(B)] > P(A \cap B')$ (eq. 2). However, $1 - P(B) = P(B')$ so that substituting in (2) we have $P(A) > P(A \cap B)/P(B')$ or $P(A|B')P(A)$, which was the point we were trying to prove. In practice things are rather more delicate than this since a simple dichotomy will not apply to the evidence.

3. This section is greatly indebted to Rouse-Ball's lively account. Ball, W. W. *Rouse (Walter William Rouse), 1850–1925: A Short Account of the History of Mathematics*, fourth edition. Macmillan, 1908.

4. That is to say, 'went shopping or on her errands'.

5. Unlike the patient he had bled.

6. A Swiss statistician will be regarded by many as being doubly cursed with tedium. No wonder the man has a chip on his shoulder.

7. Of course, the Swiss now sell cuckoo clocks to tourists but that is a different matter.

8. Galileo is of course in the absolute first rank as a physicist but, although a great mathematician, not of the same calibre as Archimedes and Lagrange or, for that matter, Euler and the Bernoullis.

9. Or possibly Frenglish.

10. See Dunham, W. *Euler, the Master of us All*. The Mathematical Association of America, 1999, p. 26.

11. See Kline, M. *Mathematical Thought from Ancient to Modern Times*. Volume 1. Oxford University edition, 1990, p. 258.

12. Sterne, L. *Tristram Shandy*. Volume VI, Chapter 23.

13. This is making the assumption that such deaths are independent. However, a person who dies from heart disease cannot die from cancer, at least not if we record a single principle cause of death, so that there may be some slight element of competition here which would invalidate the assumption of independence made. This effect is likely to be small in practice.

14. The use of a cross-over trial fixes the problem caused by differences between the proneness to seizure of different patients. There are other sources of variability over time which could still cause difficulties for this theory.

15. These and the sections that follow are based on, and heavily indebted to, Stephen Stigler's (1986) account in *The History of Statistics*. Belknap, Harvard College, Chapter 5.

16. I wish I could claim to be the originator of this excellent *bon mot*.

17. That is to say born in that which is now Belgium. The birth of the modern Belgian state dates from 1831.

18. Quetelet, A. *Physique Sociale, ou, Essai sur le Développement des Facultés de l'Homme*. Muquardt, 1869.

19. See Diamond, M. and Stone, M. Nightingale on Quetelet. *Journal of the Royal Statistical Society A* 1981; **144**: 1.

20. Quoted in Stigler (see note 16).

21. Huxley, T. H. 'The great tragedy of science – the slaying of a beautiful hypothesis by an ugly fact'. *Collected Essays (1893–1894) Biogenesis and Abiogenesis*. Macmillan, 1895.

22. This section relies heavily on the scholarly account in Hald, A. *A History of Mathematical Statistics from 1750 to 1930*. Wiley, 1988.

23. Gelfand, A. E. and Solomon, H. A study of Poisson's model for jury verdicts in criminal and civic courts. *Journal of the American Statistical Association* 1973; **68:** 271–278.

24. The probability of m or more jurors returning a verdict of guilty is the probability of $12 - m$ or fewer returning a verdict of not guilty. If the defendant is guilty an individual juror will reach this verdict with probability $1 - \theta$. Hence we need to sum the relevant binomial probabilities of a verdict of not guilty from 0 to $12 - m$. We thus have $P(\theta, m) = \sum_{x=0}^{12-m} \frac{12!}{x!(12-x)!} \theta^{12-x}(1 - \theta)^x$.

25. It is a bad policy to explain jokes, especially weak ones, but for the benefit of readers not conversant with British geography, we draw explicit attention here to the fact that there is an island in the Irish Sea called the Isle of Man.

26. Dawid, P. and Mortera, J. Coherent analysis of forensic identification evidence. *Journal of the Royal Statistical Society B* 1996; **58:** 425–443.

27. Eggleston, R. *Evidence, Proof and Probability*, 2nd edition. Weidenfeld and Nicolson, 1983.

28. Lindley, D. V. The probability approach to the treatment of uncertainty in artificial intelligence and expert systems. *Statistical Science* 1987; **2:** 17–24.

29. We can argue as follows. Consider the probability that there are X further suspects *and* that the number of suspects is more than one. We can write this as $P(X \cap X \geq 1)$, which by the rules for joint probabilities is equal to $P(X)P(X \geq 1 \mid X)$. Now if $X = 0$, the second term is simply 0. On the other hand, if $X \geq 1$ the second term is obviously 1. Therefore, the joint probability is either 0 or $P(X)$. However, by our rules for conditional probability $P(X \mid X \geq 1) = P(X \cap X \geq 1)/P(X \geq 1)$, which is therefore equal to $P(X)/P(X \geq 1)$.

30. The story of breast implant litigation is admirably recounted in Marcia Angell's book, *Science on Trial* (Norton, 1996) to which this account is indebted and from which this quotation is taken (p. 29).

31. Tugwell, P., Wells, G., Peterson, J., Welch, V., Page, J., Davison, C., McGowan, J., Ramroth, D. and Shea, B. Do silicone breast implants cause rheumatologic disorders? A systematic review for a court-appointed national science panel. *Arthritis and Rheumatism* 2001; **44:** 2477–2484.

32. Janowsky, E. C., Kupper, L. L. and Hulka, B. S. Meta-analyses of the relation between silicone breast implants and the risk of connective-tissue diseases. *New England Journal of Medicine* 2000; **342:** 781–790.

33. Tugwell et al. p. 2478.

34. Based on Figure 2 of Chapter III in Hulka, B. (principal author) *Epidemiological Analysis of Silicone Breast Implants and Connective Tissue Diseases*. Report from National Science Panel, 1998, available at http://www.fjc.gov/BREIMLIT/SCIENCE/report.htm.

35. Hulka, B. *Silicone Breast Implants in Relation to Connective Tissue Diseases and Immunologic Dysfunction*. Summary of Report of National Science Panel.

36. Hennekens, C. H., Lee, I. M., Cook, N. R., Hebert, P. R., Karlson, E. W., LaMotte, F., Manson, J. E. and Buring, J. E. Self-reported breast implants and connective-tissue

diseases in female health professionals. A retrospective cohort study. *Journal of the American Medical Association* 1996; **275**: 616–621.

37. Leontes, Act II, Scene I.
38. I am one who regards Bart as being of more cultural importance than Barthes.
39. Act III, Scene II.
40. This is in Chapter 7 of his wise and witty novel, *Coming from Behind*.

Notes to Chapter 11

1. The statistician, of course, is frequently female.
2. http://www.epolitix.com/default.asp.
3. However, not entirely unnoticed, since my account here is based on a BBC Worldwide Monitoring note of 2 May 2002.
4. This account of Lancaster's life is based on the obituary of 14 March 2002, by Paul, John and Rick Lancaster and Eugene Seneta in the *Sydney Morning Herald*.
5. Simone Manteuil-Brutlag, Interview with Dr. Margaret A. Burgess, http://cmgm. stanford.edu/biochem118/.
6. Webster, W. S. Teratogen update: congenital rubella. *Teratology* 1998; **58**: 13–23.
7. *Encyclopaedia Britannica*.
8. Lancaster, H. O. *Expectations of Life*. Springer, 1990, p. 147.
9. Lancaster, H. O. *Expectations of Life*. Springer, 1990.
10. Ibid, p. 139.
11. Pain, S. Dead man's leg. *New Scientist*, 6 July 2002, pp. 54–55.
12. Stocks, P. Measles and whooping-cough incidence before and during the dispersal of 1939–1940. *Journal of the Royal Statistical Society* 1942; **105**: 259–291.
13. Lancaster, H. O. *Expectations of Life*. Springer, 1990, p. 142. Lancaster's data are taken from Stocks (see note 12).
14. Bartlett, M S. Measles periodicity and community size. *Journal of the Royal Statistical Society A* 1957; **120**: 48–71.
15. This account is based on Petlola, H. et al. The elimination of indigenous measles, mumps, and rubella from Finland by a 12-year, two-dose vaccination program. *New England Journal of Medicine* 1994; **331**: 1397–1402.
16. These figures are based on Petlola, H. et al. 1994. However, as we have seen, we should be a little careful with such figures since the annual cases fluctuate considerably from year to year.
17. Mumps is also called infectious parotitis and the combined vaccine was sometimes referred to as MPR.
18. This section has benefited greatly from the helpful paper by Thomas, D. Rh., King, J., Evans, M. R. and Salmon, R. L. Uptake of measles containing vaccines in the measles, mumps and rubella second dose catch-up programme in Wales. *Communicable Disease and Public Health* 1998; **1**: 44–47.
19. Anderson, R. M. and May, R. M. *Infectious Diseases of Humans: Dynamics and Control*. Oxford University Press, 1991.
20. Wakefield, A. J., Murch, S. H., Anthony, A., Linnell, J., Casson, D. M., Malik, M., Berelowitz., M., Dhillon, A. P., Thomson, M. A., Harvey, P., Valentine, A., Davies, S. E. and Walker-Smith, J. A. Ileal-lymphoid-nodular hyperplasia, non-specific colilitis and pervasive developmental disorder in children. *Lancet* 1998; **351**: 637–641.
21. In June 2003 Mr Justice Sumner decided in favour of the fathers and in July 2003 the Court of Appeal upheld his judgement.

22. Taylor, B. et al. Autism and measles, mumps, and rubella vaccine: no epidemiological evidence for causal association. *The Lancet* 1999; **353**: 2026–2029.

23. Farrington, P. Relative incidence estimation from case series for vaccine safety evaluation. *Biometrics* 1995; **51**: 228–235.

24. See Small, H. *Florence Nightingale Avenging Angel.* St. Edmundsbury Press, 1998, for a fascinating account of Nightingale's statistical epiphany and Farr's role in guiding her.

25. Anderson, R. M. and May, R. M. 1991. *Infectious Diseases of Humans: Dynamics and Control.* Oxford University Press, 1991, p. 327.

26. Gehan, E. A. and Lemak, N. A. *Statistics in Medical Research, Developments in Clinical Trials.* Plenum, 1994, p. 125.

27. Meldrum, M. 'A calculated risk': the Salk polio vaccine field trials of 1954. *British Medical Journal* 1998; **317**: 1233–1236.

28. Salk Polio Vaccine Commemoration, Thomas Francis Jr. and the polio vaccine field trials, Historical Center for the Health Sciences, University of Michigan. 100 Simpson Memorial Institute/0725, 102 Observatory, Ann Arbor, MI 48109-0725. Available on-line at http://www.med.umich.edu/HCHS/articles/PolioExhibit/Francis.html.

29. Based on Bland, M. *An Introduction to Medical Statistics*, third edition. Oxford University Press, 2000.

30. See for example Hutchinson, T. A., Dawid, A. P., Spiegelhalter, D. J., Cowell, R. G. and Roden, S. Computerized aids for probabilistic assessment of drug safety I and II. *Drug Information Journal* 1991; **25**: 29–39, 41–48.

31. Quoted by BBC News on http://news.bbc.co.uk/1/hi/health/2093003.stm.

32. Hardin, G. The tragedy of the commons. In Hardin, G. *Population, Evolution and Birth Control*, second edition. WH Freeman and Co., 1969.

33. In Swiss-German my surname, Senn, means, 'a herdsman of the Alps', and I have a natural prejudice in favour of stories and metaphors involving such persons.

34. Rossi, C. Bruno de Finetti: the mathematician, the statistician, the economist, the forerunner. *Statistics in Medicine* 2001; **20**: 3651–3666.

35. The prize was awarded in 1997 to Scholes and Merton for two separate articles published in 1973. Black, who was Scholes's co-author, died in 1995 and so did not receive the prize.

36. Shafer, G. and Vovk, V. *Probability and Finance. It's Only a Game.* Wiley, 2001.

37. Cited by Menand, L. *The Metaphysical Club.* Farrar, Strauss and Giroux, 2001, p. 346.

38. Cox, D. R. Deming lecture to the Joint Statistical Meeting, New York, August 2002.

Index